VACCINE INJURED CHILDREN

21st Century Tragedy

Treatment, Prevention, Reasons

Dr Isaac Golden

2023 4th Edition
2019 3rd Edition
2010 2nd Edition
2008 1st Edition

Vaccine Injured Children: 21st Century Tragedy. Treatment, Prevention, Reasons

Dr Isaac Golden PhD, DHom, ND, BEc (Hon)
Deputy Chair and Research Consultant, Ethics Committee, National Institute of Integrative Medicine, Melbourne.
Principal, Aurum Healing Centre, Cherokee, Victoria.
Director, Australasian College of Hahnemannian Homoeopathy.
Director, Homoeopathy International Online College.
Honorary Research Fellow, School of Science, Federation University, 2013-2016.
President, Australian Homoeopathic Association (Victoria), 1992-1998.
Australian Homoeopathic Association, Distinguished Service Award, 13.3.1999.

Inquiries: Postal: P.O. Box 695, Gisborne. Victoria. Australia. 3437.
Phone: (03) 5427 0880
E-Mail: admin@homstudy.net

Web Pages: www.homstudy.net (link to different pages)

 Photo by Richard Stachmann on Unsplash

ISBN: 978-0-9578726–6-0
National Library, Canberra (02) 6262 1434

Other Publications by the Author:

Immunisation Options for Parents Who Care 2015
ISBN 13:978-1508741992

The Complete Practitioners Manual of Homoeoprophylaxis. 2017
ISBN 13:978-1478388050

Vaccination & Homoeoprophylaxis? - A Review of Risks and Alternatives. 7th ed. 2010.
ISBN 978-0-9578726-4-6

Homœoprophylaxis - A Practical and Philosophical Review. 4th ed. 2007
ISBN 0 - 646 - 19529 - 8

Homœoprophylaxis – A Fifteen Year Clinical Study. 2004.
ISBN 0 - 9578 - 7263 - 1

Homœoprophylaxis – A Ten Year Clinical Study. 1997
ISBN 0 – 646 – 32054 – 8

Australian Homoeopathic Home Prescriber - Part 1. 3rd ed. 2007
ISBN 0 - 646 - 15057 - X

Australian Homoeopathic Home Prescriber - Part 2. 2001
ISBN 0 – 9578726 – 0 – 7

Australian Homoeopathic Home Prescriber - Part 3. 2006
ISBN 0 – 9578726 – 5 - 3

Homoeopathic Body-System Prescribing - A Practical Workbook of Sector Remedies, 2nd ed. 2002 ISBN 0 - 646 - 27292 - 6

Homoeopathic Treatment of the Energy Bodies. 2002
ISBN 0 – 9578726 – 1 - 5

Preface

2023

Between the 2019 edition and 2023 the world has been forced to endure 3 years of madness, and sadness.

The pain will last for decades and was largely unnecessary. It was imposed on the world by people who ranged from ignorant to corrupt. "Experts" who lied. Politicians who abrogated their responsibility to those who elected them - to you and me. Journalists who relegated themselves to being unquestioning outlets for the deceitful "spin" of the pharmaceutical drug cartels, and the cartels became the real beneficiaries of Covid 19.

The truth was available for those who wanted to hear it, but most people didn't want to hear. In this edition I will add a little more inconvenient truth - some data I have been collecting regarding the treatment of vaccine injury from Covid "vaccines".

But the two major goals of the 2023 edition are (1) to update my data to 31.12.22, and (2) to try to make the book more readable. The second goal has led me to try to simplify some of the Tables, at times by creating a new Table to spread the data over two and make each easier to understand. For example, I simplified Table 10 and put some of the information into Table 10.5.

I have kept the idea of answering four major questions, but have split the total content into four Parts:
Part 1: Introduction and Background
Part 2: Results
Part 3: Conclusions
Part 4: Resources and Appendices

The idea is that if a reader wishes to go straight to the results of my treatment programs, they can skip Part 1 and go straight to Part 2.

I have kept alternating data with cases as in previous editions and added two new cases at the end.

I hope these changes will make this 4th Edition both more current and more accessible.

2019

I changed the lead title from *Vaccine Damaged Children* to *Vaccine Injured Children* because of feedback from a group of mothers whose children had been adversely affected by vaccines. They all asked for the word "injured" to be used in preference to "damaged", it made sense, and I have respected their wishes. I added "21st Century Tragedy" to the title because that is what this is, and what history will (long after I have departed this embodiment) show it to be.

I have added new cases, updated old ones, and totally revised my own data with the latest figures collected to 31.12.18 and reanalysed in 2019.

I considered whether to completely change the structure of the book, but decided to keep the content centred on 4 questions:

1. Do vaccines cause injury?

2. What are the symptoms of vaccine injury?
3. Can we prevent vaccine injury?
4. How do we treat vaccine injury?

After all, the answers to these questions are what this journey is all about. But I have renumbered sections within each Question/Chapter to hopefully make finding relevant material easier.

Over the last 10 years there has been an unfortunate increase in attacks on parents who ask thoughtful questions about vaccination, and even parents who relate their own deeply distressing experiences with vaccine injury. National media are typically aggressively hostile to anyone who asks serious and reasonable questions about vaccination. The media refuse to examine and publish evidence about vaccine injury.

And this has all occurred while government organisations lie to us about a range of health issues, including vaccine injury, as exposed by insiders such as Dr William Thompson from the CDC (Centre for Disease Control – the peak USA organisation regulating vaccination) who revealed that CDC researchers deliberately concealed a link between vaccination and autism. And that a CDC funded researcher, Paul Thorsen, who co-authored articles refuting the vaccination-autism link is facing criminal charges for fraud, as well as accusations of research fraud.

We need change, urgently. Too much damage has already been done. Too many children and their families harmed. Too many lies told.

I am not anti-vaccination. I believe that every parent has the right to use vaccines to protect their children against potentially serious infectious diseases. But I also believe every parent has the right to know the truth about all immunisation options, and full details regarding the safety and effectiveness of all options, and thus be able to make fully informed decisions.

My hope is that this small book assists not only parents of vaccine injured children, but also parents of yet-to-be-immunised children. I also hope this book will become a valuable resource for practitioners of any modality who are called upon to recognise and treat vaccine injury.

2008

My first experience with a vaccine injured child occurred in the late 1970's, with my own daughter. This is why I have never needed anyone to convince me that vaccine injury is a reality.

It is also why I immediately mistrust anyone who claims that vaccines are completely safe. Apart from the fact that the orthodox medical literature has many references to vaccine injury, and apart from the fact that vaccine inserts acknowledge that vaccines can cause injury, and apart from the fact that some Governments have paid out hundreds of millions of dollars in vaccine injury compensation (the USA alone over 4 billion to date), many "scientists" continue to claim that they are safe.

Before I studied homoeopathic medicine, I used to follow the advice I was given by doctors. To this day I don't know whether the doctors who convinced me to continue vaccinating my daughter, even after her first adverse reactions, intentionally deceived me or sincerely believed that the vaccines were not responsible for her health disorders. I suspect the latter, but either way I was misled in my ignorance by their ignorance, and my daughter suffered.

Once I studied homoeopathic medicine, I discovered that it offered a safe and comparably effective alternative to vaccination. Thus, began what has ended up being a major part of my professional life – the development and statistical analysis of a long-term preventative (immunisation) program that parents can use instead of vaccination - if they choose. Following from this work has been an active involvement in the treatment of vaccine injured children.

This is not all I do by any means, but nothing else is more important.

The tragedy that vaccine injury inflicts not only upon the injured child, but the whole family, can be immense. And the real tragedy is that it is completely avoidable.

Time has taught me that most GP's are basically sincere people who want to help others. Some are arrogant because they are imbued with that attitude in medical school. Most are fixed in their ideas regarding the superiority of their methods over all others, leaving them ignorant of alternatives. This is a great shame, because I am sure that if all GP's were truly aware of the injury they are pushing onto children, that many more would moderate their vaccination practices – a few do publicly, and more do so privately. And maybe those politicians who are not influenced by Pharma "donations" would take notice and write appropriate legislation.

In 2008 and again in 2010, 2012 and 2014 I saw firsthand a system of public health that encourages GPs to use the best interventions for their patients from all healing systems. I visited Cuba, firstly at their invitation and then on my own initiative to study their massive homeopathic immunisation programs involving over 2,200,000 people in 2007 and 2008 against leptospirosis and then over 9,800,000 people in 2010 against Swine Flu.

I saw their hospitals where multi-skilled doctors were doing marvellous work using acupuncture, herbal medicines, homeopathy, nutrition etc alongside modern western techniques. Not only were their results impressive, but they also achieved improved results at a fraction of the cost of using only western drug-based approaches. More importantly full treatment was available for all residents, not just the wealthy or the insured.

I hope and pray that a new generation of doctors might arise whose eyes and hearts are open to all the wonderful healing methods God has provided.

My assumption of good intentions does not extend to multinational pharmaceutical companies. I have no doubt that they know exactly what they are imposing on our children. The fact that vaccines may cause chronic health problems in many children simply means that they make even greater profits in the chemical treatment of the consequent diseases. And that is the only thing that matters to these companies - profits.

If they can happily dump rejected drugs on third world countries, if they can permanently silence critics, if they can distort the research on which medical decisions and national legislation are based, if they can spend literally billions of dollars annually to buy influence in the highest levels of Government, if they can finance "skeptics" to attack natural options, and after all that distribute harmful chemicals which they know cause chronic health problems - it is no more than their daily business. They are organisations of darkness.

But this book is about children whose lives have been changed, some slightly, some massively, by vaccines. This book is about how to recognise vaccine injury, and some methods to treat it. It also recommends how to prevent vaccine injury.

It is a book for parents of vaccine injured children. I hope it will be a positive book which can bring you some hope in what is for some a life of daily suffering. It is also a book which I hope will be helpful and supportive to practitioners from all modalities.

It is a factual book. It intentionally does not try to be emotive. Emotions are not needed to make the points needed to make, just facts.

We will ask, and answer, four basic questions:

1. Do vaccines cause injury?
2. What are the symptoms of vaccine injury?
3. How can we prevent vaccine injury?
4. How do we treat vaccine injury?

The answers to these questions are supported by many facts, figures, and case examples. Hopefully this information will allow you to become much better informed about all aspects of vaccine injury, and give you some strategies as to how to help those who have been vaccine injured.

Between the Chapters covering the above four questions are case examples. These cases are presented to illustrate the practical aspects of the treatment of vaccine injury. A final Chapter will present a further group of cases. The important thing to know in treatment is that every patient is different, and one protocol does not fit everyone. Flexibility and the willingness to change a "typical" treatment program according to the individual patient's reactions are essential.

The real tragedy is that in too many cases, severe vaccine injury cannot be reversed. However appropriate homoeopathic treatment is always worth trying. As the cases show, it is also possible to see amazing results which can change a person's life for the better.

I am a homoeopath, so I have not attempted to provide detailed information on nutritional, TCM, chiropractic and other treatments. On its own, homoeopathy can provide amazing results, but the patient's complete lifestyle including diet and supplementation is always important. A supportive family environment is always significant. But sometimes even the best treatments don't work. This is where homoeopathy can show its value, as it can remove "layers" of disorder in a way that other excellent modalities cannot. A final Appendix provides a simple introduction to homoeopathy.

Whether you are a person suffering from vaccine injury, a parent of a child who has been vaccine injured, or a practitioner of any modality including orthodox medicine, my sincere hope it that this little book will assist you in your decision making.

Acknowledgements

I would like to thank Dr Chris Turville for the contributions he made to my work on homœoprophylaxis and on the treatment of vaccine injured children during 2008. Chris is a statistician in the School of Information Technology and Mathematical Sciences at University of Ballarat. I greatly appreciate his professionalism and support in this work.
I would also like to thank my daughter (remedial therapist and homoeopath) Leiah Sophia Golden for her review of the draft of the revised 2010 edition.

A Note on the Cover

Whenever I work with vaccine injured children, and see what a tragedy it is that these children and their families to have to suffer so much, I am continually asking myself – WHY – why won't the medical people acknowledge and correct what is happening here?

This is also a question many parents ask me – if we have all this information, WHY do the health authorities still allow such dreadful injury to occur?

WHY?

The answer will reveal the failings of generations of men and women whom we trusted to care for us and for our children. There is no nice way to say this, and history will judge accordingly.

Table of Contents

Index of Tables and Figures

Definitions

Antigen – a substance that the body recognises as being not of itself, thus provoking an immune response.

Antibody – an immunoglobulin (one of 5 classes of protein) produced to protect against an antigen.

The **Effectiveness** of a homoeopathic preventative program is the proportion of those using the program who did not acquire the targeted disease, to the total number of persons using the program. Where possible, the figure for effectiveness is refined by identifying those users of the program who were exposed to the targeted disease, and using that total in the proportion.

The **Genus Epidemicus** is the homoeopathic remedy chosen during an outbreak of an infectious disease that best matches the common symptom picture of the disease. The remedy is selected after analysing the symptoms of several patients with the disease.

Homœoprophylaxis (HP) is the use of homoeopathically prepared potentised substances in a systematic manner to prevent the development of the characteristic symptoms of infectious diseases.

An **Isode** is a remedy prepared from the patient's OWN diseased material, e.g., a remedy prepared from a whooping-cough patient's own sputum.

Immunisation is taken to mean any method that reduces the likelihood of the recipient acquiring a targeted infectious disease if exposed to the disease.

The **Law of Similars** states that a substance that can cause a group of symptoms in a healthy person can remove a group of **similar** symptoms in a sick person.

A **Nosode** is a homoeopathic preparation (potency) of diseased tissue, e.g., a remedy prepared from the sputum of several patients with whooping cough.

Potentisation is the method used in homoeopathy to prepare remedies. The original material is subjected to a series of dilutions and succussions (violent shaking of the diluting medium against a firm surface), or triturations (grinding of insoluble substances).

Provings are controlled experiments where doses of the substance being tested (usually in potentised form) are given to healthy volunteers, who record new symptoms produced by taking the substance. The Master Prover (the person supervising the proving) then extracts those symptoms that are common to several provers, and this information is entered into the Materia Medica.

Succussion is the process used in the preparation of homoeopathic remedies in liquid form where the container holding the medicinal solution is repeatedly shaken firmly with vertical movements against a firm surface thus violently agitating the medicinal solution.

Trituration is the process used in the preparation of homoeopathic remedies in solid form where the active substance and a medicinally neutral powder, often sugar crystals prepared from maize or milk, are ground together using a mortar and pestle. Usually, trituration is used only until the mixture is soluble.

Vaccination is defined as the administration, usually orally or by injection, of attenuated antigenic material together with preservatives and adjuvants to stimulate the production of antibodies in the recipient.

The **Vital Force** is defined by homoeopaths as a person's self-balancing (healing) energy that is present from birth, and which acts to maintain homoeostasis on the mental, emotional, and physical levels of the person's being.

Overview 2019 (and 2023)

1. We know that vaccines may cause injury.
2. We know that health authorities know this, yet laws are made to protect and reward the perpetrators.
3. Anyone who simply questions the balance between the risks and benefits of vaccination, or asks for more research, is demonised in the media as being "anti-vaxx".
4. Parents who deeply care about their children's health are accused of being thoughtless, and of putting others at risk.
5. There is no debate about these life-and-death issues, there are different sides shouting at each other.
6. Behind this, the people who direct the pharmaceutical cartels remain unjudged, unaccountable, and untouchable.
7. As well, some unethical researchers, practitioners, bureaucrats, media owners and politicians become wealthy, yet immune to consequences.
8. Simple, honest, open discussion is banned and has been replaced by anger, hostility, ignorance, and confusion.

We are in a negative place where safe, inexpensive, proven choices are attacked, and unsafe, expensive, health-destroying options are promoted. **Medical systems have become about disease management. Wealth creation for a few has replaced health creation for the majority.**

We have poisoned our environment, and we are poisoning our people. Are we so stupid that we cannot see this? Are we so apathetic that we will not challenge this? If the answers are "yes" then our path is decided.

Is this really what you want for your children's children?

PART 1: Introduction and Background

Question 1: Do Vaccines Cause Injury?

1.1 Vaccine Injury

Possibly the simplest way to resolve this question is to (i) examine the amounts of compensation for vaccine injury paid by governments around the world who acknowledge vaccine injury, and (ii) see what vaccine manufacturers say in vaccine inserts.

If vaccines did not cause injury, then these compensation payments, now exceeding 4 billion dollars in the USA alone, would not have been made. In fact, they represent the tip of a huge "iceberg" of chronic vaccine injury (for example, the UK scheme requires 80% or greater disability).

In Australia there is a culture among most GPs to refuse to acknowledge vaccine injury. In a case I saw in March 2008, 6 teenage girls from the same school were immediately and seriously adversely affected by the HPV vaccine. My patient was one of the girls. She developed uncontrollable trembling of the extremities 15 minutes after the vaccine, which was still present a week later when she first consulted me. She had seen five doctors and specialists, all of whom refused to acknowledge the possibility of vaccine injury and put her and her classmates' reactions down to hysteria. Similar experiences are met with similar denials from doctors.

Unlike the Australian government, the following 19 Governments have some form of vaccine injury compensation:

1960's - West Germany (since 1961), France (since 1964),
1970's – Switzerland (since 1970), Japan (since 1976), Denmark, New Zealand, Sweden, UK (since 1979) Austria

1980's - Finland, Taiwan, the Province of Quebec (since 1985), USA (since 1988),
1990's – Italy, Norway, South Korea (since 1994).
2000's – Hungary, Iceland, Slovenia.

Details were outlined in Looker C & Kelly H. No-fault compensation following adverse events attributed to vaccination: a review of international programmes. *Bulletin of the World Health Organization 2011;89:371-378. doi: 10.2471/BLT.10.081901* (accessed 17/7/19).

We shall now examine some vaccine injury compensation schemes to see the extent of potential injury.

1.2 USA Compensation Scheme

In 1988 the US Government introduced a *National Vaccine Injury Compensation Scheme* (NCVIS). The complete set of data is shown in Appendix 1. The total compensation paid to 2019 now exceeds 4 billion dollars, as shown in Table 1. A breakdown of claims by death or injury is summarised in Table 2, and a breakdown by type of vaccine is shown in Table 3 (main claims only).

The data is taken from the National Vaccine Injury Compensation Program - US Department of Health and Human Resources (now known as Health and Human Services). HRSA – Health Resources and Services Administration

It is revealing to notice that this legislation has attracted several legal firms in the USA to specialise in representing parents of vaccine injured children.

The NVICS states on a FAQ's about finding an attorney:

Q. Can NVICS help me find an attorney specializing in vaccine laws and exemptions?
A: There are a number of attorneys and law firms specializing in bringing vaccine injury claims before the U.S. Court of Claims under the National Childhood Vaccine Injury Act's Vaccine Injury Compensation Program. However, it is difficult to find a lawyer who will assist parents in filing or defending a medical, religious or conscientious belief exemption to state vaccine laws.
The federal Vaccine Injury Compensation Program (VICP) no longer provides a list of attorneys that handle vaccine injury claims on their website. However, the U.S. Court of Federal Claims provides an attorney list. The VICP also states that this information may be available from state and/or local bar associations.
When deciding on legal representation, consider the experience, success and whether or not the attorney is recognized by the VICP. If you are unsuccessful finding an attorney to represent you, you could also try the vaccine injury clinic at George Washington University – please note that students serve as the attorney (with supervision).
https://www.nvic.org/faqs/attorney-directory.aspx (accessed 16/7/19).

Table 1: NVICS Compensation Payments to 1st June 2023

	Post 1988 Claims		**Pre 1988 Claims**	
Petitions Filed	20,215 (inc. 1,290 deaths)		4,264	
	Compensatable	**Dismissed**	**Compensatable**	**Dismissed**
Petitions Decided	9,831	12,452	2,542**	
	$4,858.4m	$167.2m*	$902.52m	
Total Paid to 1st June 2023 = $5,025.7 mill. ** USD				

* - compensation not awarded, but legal fees paid
** - includes compensation, plus legal fees only

Table 2: Claims by Event (Death or Injury) to 1st June 2023

	Injury	Death	Total	Compensated	Dismissed
TOTAL	24,825	1,402	26,227	9,895	12,452

Note: the difference in figures relates to claims being processed, but not yet decided.

Table 3: Claims by Type of Vaccine to 1st June 2023 (main claims only - sorted by Claims Compensated)

Vaccines	Filed			Compe	Dismi
	Injury	Death	Total	-nsated	-ssed
Influenza	9.095	234	9,329	5,588	993
DTP	3,288	696	3,984	1,273	2,711
Tdap	1,218	8	1,226	696	154
MMR	1,048	63	1,111	432	612
Hepatitis B	751	62	813	304	449
DTaP	486	88	574	258	278
HPV	777	21	798	167	419
OPV	282	28	310	158	152
Td	241	3	244	141	80
Pneumococcal Conjugate	334	24	358	136	95
Tetanus	187	3	190	104	49
Rotavirus	117	6	123	76	33
Varicella	117	10	127	72	39
Rubella	190	4	194	71	123
Hepatitis A	145	7	152	70	45
Meningococcal	125	3	128	70	29
Measles	145	19	164	57	107
DTaP-Hep B-IPV	101	40	141	48	68
DT	69	9	78	26	52

MMR-Varicella	62	2	64	26	21
Hep A-Hep B	46	0	46	23	9
HIB	50	3	53	23	22
DTaP-IPV-HIB	53	21	74	18	41
Unspecified **	5,427	9	5,436	11	5,419
IPV	269	14	283	10	271
DTaP-HIB	11	1	12	7	4
DTP-HIB	20	8	28	7	21
DTaP-IPV	16	0	16	6	5
MR	15	0	15	6	9
Hep B-HIB	8	0	8	5	3
Nonqualified *	118	13	131	3	125
Pertussis	4	3	7	2	5
Mumps	10	0	10	1	9
DTaP-IPV-HIB-HEPB	0	0	0	0	0
Total	24,825	1,402	26,227	9,895	12,452

* Nonqualified petitions are those filed for vaccines not covered under the NVICS.
** Unspecified petitions are those submitted with insufficient information to make a determination.

Government official statistics to 1st June, 2023.
https://www.hrsa.gov/sites/default/files/hrsa/vicp/vicp-stats.pdf

* * * * * * *

1.3 UK Compensation Scheme

The UK government established a Vaccine Injury Payment Scheme in 1979. Unlike the USA situation, the UK government does not provide up to date information on the public record. Their scheme caps the maximum payout to victims.

The UK Government states that "If you're severely disabled as a result of a vaccination against certain diseases, you could get a one-off tax-free payment of £120,000. This is called a Vaccine Damage Payment." ***https://www.gov.uk/vaccine-damage-payment*** (accessed 10/6/23).

Most data available had to be drawn from the government under freedom of information claims. Hence the data in the following news-release is dated, but it is still instructive.

> BBC News Wednesday, 16 March, 2005, reported that the government has paid out £3.5m to 35 patients left disabled by vaccinations since 1997.
>
> The Department of Work and Pensions could not reveal which jabs were involved in the claims. The figure was revealed to the Evening Standard newspaper under the Freedom of Information Act.
>
> It was also revealed that a total of 917 payments have been made since the Vaccine Injury Payment Scheme was introduced in 1979.
>
> Vaccine injury payments are one-off payments to people who are able to prove that they were severely disabled as a result of a vaccination. Many thousands of claims are likely to have been made under the scheme but were unsuccessful.

More recently, the Department provided the following information under a Freedom of Information Request.

"22 March 2017

FOI 1075690

Dear Mr XXXXXXX

Thank you for your
request of 23 February 2017 under the Freedom of
Information Act (2000). Your exact request was:
"Please could you give me the following information:-
1) How many claims for Vaccine Damage Compensation have been made in the last 10 years?
2) How many of these claims were successful?"

I can confirm that the Department holds
the information you requested.
I would like to clarify that the Vaccine Damage Payment Scheme (VDP S) is not a compensation scheme, and was never
intended by Parliament to be such. It provides a one off, tax-free, lump sum payment of £120,000 for those who are
severely disabled as a result of a vaccination against those diseases listed in the Vaccine Damage Payments Act 1979 and those diseases that have been specified since 1979 by statutory instrument.
From 2007/08 to 31 January 2017, there have been a total
of 759 claims and 11 awards made. It should be noted that an award might be made in a different year to that which the claim was made. "
https://www.whatdotheyknow.com/request/391400/response/955853/attach/html/2/FOI%201075690%20Griffin%20VDPS%20claims%20v2%204.pdf.html (accessed 17/7/19).

1.4 Japanese Compensation Scheme

The Preventative Vaccine Law in Japan was amended in 1976 to provide for relief for injury in cases where unavoidable side effects result from preventative vaccination.

1977 to 1981
226 cases: 167 approved, 45 denied, 14 pending as of 1983

Reference: Data was previously available at http://www.nap.edu/openbook.php?record_id=599&page=180, but this reference appears to have been withdrawn.

An article discussing the withdrawal of HPV vaccination in Japan and confusion in the compensation scheme is:
Yuji K and Nakada H. Compensation programs after withdrawal of the recommendation for HPV vaccine in Japan. *Human Vaccines & Immunotherapeutics.* 2016. 12(5);1321-1324. (accessed 28/8/23).

The budget for 88 certified claims in 2019 was $US10.8 million.
Reference: Fujiwara Y, Onda Y, Hayashi S. No fault compensation schemes for COVID-19 medical products. *The Lancet*, 2021. **397**(10286);1707-1708.

More recently, Japanese authorities will pay a bereaved family a lump sum of 44.2 million yen should one of them die after taking the Covid-19 jab.

The figure, which is the equivalent to around £295,350, is the highest one-off fee that could be paid out by the Japanese government in the case of an adverse reaction to the Coronavirus jab.

Families may also receive a 5,056,800 yen (£33,700) annual payment should someone suffer a long-term disability that requires care because of taking the jab, while funeral costs in the eventuality of any death would also be covered up to 209,000 yen (£1395).

https://www.ladbible.com/news/news-japanese-families-will-receive-44-million-yen-if-covid-vaccine-kills-20210224 (accessed 28/8/23).

1.5 Vaccine Manufacturers Inserts

The vaccine manufacturers themselves acknowledge a range of possible adverse events, showing the stupidity of claims by ill-informed politicians and others that "vaccines are completely safe". A few examples are now given.

Infanrix Hexa: Made by GSK to protect against Diphtheria, Pertussis, Tetanus, Hib, Hep B and Polio. The 38 page PRODUCT MONOGRAPH is available at https://ca.gsk.com/media/537989/infanrix-hexa.pdf (accessed 15/7/19).
Readers can draw their own conclusions, but it is clear that there are relatively few safety studies (one with 267 subjects which lasted 8 days only and used another vaccine as a control, one with 16,000 subjects which was not clearly referenced and with no study details such as duration or control).
Part III CONSUMER INFORMATION at the end of the monograph listed a range of common and less common adverse events with the disclaimer "This is not a complete list of side effects".

MMRV (ProQuad): Made by Merck to protect against Measles, Mumps, Rubella and Varicella (Chicken Pox). Technical details are available from FDA at https://www.fda.gov/media/75203/download (accessed 15/7/19).
Most quoted studies compared reactions with ProQuad with other vaccines like MMR II and VARIVAX (a common statistical trick used to lessen the apparent extent of adverse reactions that would be revealed if compared with an inactive placebo). A long list of possible side effects is given on pages 11-14. The risk of shedding is given on page 4.

Gardasil: Made by Merck to protect against some strains of Human Papiloma Virus. Technical details are available from FDA at https://www.fda.gov/media/74350/download (accessed 15/7/19). A range of studies are quoted, but of most interest is on page 10 where it stated:

"**6.2 Postmarketing Experience** The following adverse events have been spontaneously reported during post-approval use of GARDASIL. Because these events were reported voluntarily from a population of uncertain size, it is not possible to reliably estimate their frequency or to establish a causal relationship to vaccine exposure.

Blood and lymphatic system disorders: Autoimmune hemolytic anemia, idiopathic thrombocytopenic purpura, lymphadenopathy.

Respiratory, thoracic and mediastinal disorders: Pulmonary embolus.

Gastrointestinal disorders: Nausea, pancreatitis, vomiting.

General disorders and administration site conditions: Asthenia, chills, death, fatigue, malaise.

Immune system disorders: Autoimmune diseases, hypersensitivity reactions including anaphylactic/anaphylactoid reactions, bronchospasm, and urticaria.

Musculoskeletal and connective tissue disorders: Arthralgia, myalgia.

Nervous system disorders: Acute disseminated encephalomyelitis, dizziness, Guillain-Barré syndrome, headache, motor neuron disease, paralysis, seizures, syncope (including syncope associated with tonicclonic movements and other seizure-like activity) sometimes resulting in falling with injury, transverse myelitis.

Infections and infestations: cellulitis.

Vascular disorders: Deep venous thrombosis."

It is revealing to compare the above lists with the VAERS data base noted earlier. The point being made here though is that it is simply inaccurate to claim that vaccines are completely safe as official inserts and documentation show this not to be the case. This is not saying that vaccines are more or less unsafe than the diseases they are designed to prevent - that is a different discussion.

1.5 Concluding comments

More information about vaccine injury is listed in Section 2, however the information presented above from just a few countries and from just a few vaccine inserts shows unambiguously that vaccines can cause injury. This finding is completely unsurprising to any person who seeks information, despite the increasing attempts of Google, Facebook, health bureaucracies and the mainstream media to suppress information regarding vaccine injury. As said earlier, the above information represents the tip of a very large iceberg.

In fact, there is a glaring absence in medical journals of published research on the long-term impact of vaccination on the overall wellbeing of recipients. If the research has been done, then the results have been withheld. If the research has not been done, then parents have every reason to ask why not.

It is inexcusable to impose a medical procedure on millions of children and not thoroughly investigate the long-term potential for injury to the overall wellbeing of recipients.

We have a hidden epidemic of injury. We know that the incidence of chronic illness in "developed" countries is huge. For example, in Australia official Australian Bureau of Statistics figures show that 40% of all children aged 14 years or less have at least one chronic illness. The cause of this disturbingly high figure is not given, and of course vaccination is not the only possible cause, but the above information suggests it is highly likely to be a significant contributing factor.

Parents deserve honesty from health officials. Politicians need objective and accurate advice from their bureaucrats. Patients deserve the best treatment from their medical practitioners. Doctors need accurate information during their training in medical schools.

What no one needs is the economic power and influence of pharmaceutical giants corrupting our health system - from their control of medical research with its consequent influence over medical training, to their purchase of influence at Government level, to their domination of mass media and journalism through multi-million-dollar advertising expenditure.

The negative influence of the pharmaceutical industry has been documented in great detail by researchers at Harvard University. The information is available for free and should be required reading for all medical students and politicians, as well as health bureaucrats.

The Harvard analysis comprised a symposium on **Institutional Corruption and Pharmaceutical Policy** published in the *Journal of Law, Medicine & Ethics*, Vol. 41, No. 3 (2013). All symposium articles are accessible through the Edmond J. Safra Center for Ethics website through the following link: https://ethics.harvard.edu/news/jlme-issue-institutional-corruption-and-pharmaceutical-industry (accessed 31/8/23).

I published an article in 2018 summarising these reviews, as well as detailing the incidence of chronic disease in Australia (figures which would be similar in many "developed" countries).

Golden I. Confronting our Diseased Healthcare System: some causes and cures. *Similia*. Dec 2018. **30**(2); 9-13. Available online at www.healthaustraliaparty.com.au/news-articles-resources/topic/

So the answer is "yes – vaccines may cause injury". This does not on its own mean that vaccination does not have benefits, and there needs to be an honest comparison of benefits and risks, and a truthful evaluation of alternatives.

The root cause of vaccine injury rests with people and organisations that know the truth, and not only refuse to inform parents and politicians, but in fact conceal the truth through every means possible

Cases: Two Cases of Multiple Layers of Vaccine Injury

1.6 A brief outline of the homoeopathic method

Some readers will not be familiar with homoeopathic medicine, and for this reason I have included a brief outline of the homoeopathic method in Appendix 6 so that you will better understand the following case material. Please feel free to turn to it at any time to assist your understanding of the reasons for the method used in the following cases.

The explanation is taken largely from the third booklet in my home prescribing series, *Australian Homoeopathic Home Prescriber: Part 3 – A Simple Introduction to Homoeopathic Medicine* (2006).

One point to note is that homoeopathic remedies are prescribed in different strengths or potencies. The normal range is 30, 200, 1,000 (or M), 10,000 (or 10M), 50M, 100M (or CM), 500M, 1,000M (or MM).

Thus, you will find each prescription showing the remedy name and the potency. For example, "DPT M" means the M or 1,000th potency of the triple antigen (DPT) vaccine.

Actual names are of course not given in the cases in this book, however the dates are correct. Because I choose to live in somewhat remote areas, I do a lot of phone and now internet follow-ups, which are the dates shown between the first and subsequent consultations.

In some of the cases I have made comments explaining the use of certain remedies. I have put these personal comments in italics.

1.7 Case 135 – "Sam"

Overview: Sam's case illustrates how a vaccine (in this case the MMR vaccine) can create a "layer" of disturbance (autistic type symptoms) on top of another level of disturbance caused by the DPT vaccine (aggression, ADHD type symptoms). The MMR potency helped to remove the most recent layer first revealing the deeper layer, and then the DPT potency worked on the ADHD type layer.
Sam had one of the most dramatic reactions to a vaccine potency which I have ever seen (a massive expulsion of worms). We spent most of the time waiting for each dose to do its job, and the improvement continues to be dramatic.
This is the longest case in the book which has been updated in the 2010 Revision. It has currently been going for 2½ years, but shows what is possible when parents give sufficient time for remedies to complete their work.

27.11.07. 1st consultation.
Male, 3 years of age.
For the first 12 months of his life, Sam was a happy boy who mixed well with people. Then on 25/5/05 had the following vaccines: MMR, Meningitis A & C, Hib and Hep B.
He had a reaction, including sweating and a temperature. He was not able to move his arm for 2 days. The doctor said he had hit a muscle.

A couple of months later he was very sick for 6 weeks, with vomiting for 2 weeks and diarrhoea for 4 weeks. He refused food and became very hyperactive.
After that time he would improve for 4-5 days, then have vomiting for 10 days. After some time that pattern finished.

However, he was never free of diarrhoea.

He was NEVER HAPPY, whined a lot, avoided cuddles and would play up. Slept a lot. Was both hyperactive and fatigued.
He stopped talking (would point and cry). Some words came back around 2y/o. FOOD SENSITIVITY.
At 2 y/o they saw a paediatrician who did a lot of tests which showed an elevated white cell count (Dr said he had an infection). Lumps in the back of his neck.

NOW: parents took him off formula 4 weeks ago and the diarrhoea stopped, but now he is constipated with a motion every 3rd day. Less hyperactivity, but REALLY BAD AGGRESSION. Will lash out at his parents.

The Doctor diagnosed him with PERVASIVE DELAYED DEVELOPMENT AUTISTIC SPECTRUM. He also said that Sam would not be able to go to a normal school. The Doctors want him to be officially diagnosed with Aspergers/Autism. They also said that his mother should see a psychiatrist.

Now, he lines things up. He is very upset if strangers look at him. When he is upset, he is much better if placed in a bath. Better if his mother presses her hand of his stomach which calms him. Sam will press her hand hard into his stomach. He is also better in a car.

Rx. (1) MMR M fortnightly.

3.12.07 Sam EXPELLED A MASSIVE NUMBER OF WORMS ++ (he had never done this before). Swollen eyes, dribbling, cough, emotionally fragile. His cheek swelled (like occurred following the injection).
5.12.07 High fever. Better in general.
7.12.07 High temperature with a cold and a cough.

11.1.08 (2nd consultation) Has only had one dose of the MMR M. Very significant reaction. Now has much better eye contact. His eyes are

clearer than before. Now he won't stop talking to others. Less compulsive, but still lines up chairs when in a different environment, and still has a fascination with water.
Now, he is more defiant. He wants to get his own way and wants to be in control. He will cry to get sympathy. He will either (i) talk a lot, (ii) get his own way, or (iii) try to keep changing things.
He is not physically aggressive but will have an outburst every now and then. Is much better with other children but needs to be on his terms. He wants to be accepted. Is better with older children.
His parents gave him a dose of worm tablets from the chemist 3 weeks ago. He became more aggressive.
Sam's dad said that his hyperactivity began at 7 months of age following the DPT vaccine.
Rx. Hold the (1) MMR M, and use (2) Cina 30 for worms if necessary.

7.2.08 (3rd consultation)
(2) Cina 30 helped Sam to sleep through the night. Still has not repeated the (1) MMR M.
His speech is now much better.
He is very dependent on his mum at the moment.
In general, better in the morning, then around 2pm becomes fatigued, then cried, then becomes agitated. Then around 7pm becomes hyperactive.
He went to kinder. Was OK if left alone, but unsettled if a teacher disturbed him.
Food: craves cheese, sweets, ice cream. Very hard to get Sam to eat other foods.

Rx. Give a second dose of (1) MMR M. Use (3) Cina 200 weekly as required.

15.2.08 Face became swollen again after MMR M. Now face is better but he has become very disturbed after attending an early invention program recommended by doctors.

4.3.08 Is improving, even the people at the intervention program see a change.

18.4.08 (4th consultation). Things are good at the moment. He had a single tablet of (1) MMR M without any reaction, then a dose of 2 tablets without a definite reaction.
However, his general health and his language have both improved. He is singing!!
His mother believes that he had now come out of the autistic state.
He is interacting with people, talking, outgoing.
She now believes he has moved into a more ADHD type of behaviour where he can have meltdowns which are worse when he is frustrated.
He will also become very determined and fiddles with hands.
He also is becoming intensely interested in things around him. He will run off, and not sit still. His voice is now very loud.
He is taking his clothes off and runs. He is annoyed by clothing, especially by clothing around his neck, and by socks and shoes.
Some fear of the dark. Constant burping with hiccoughs.

Rx. (4) DPT M, (5) Lach 200, (6) Giardia 200. The remedies to be used as directed depending on symptom changes *(note: the remedies will be spaced apart, and only used if directed by myself. The patient lives hours from my clinic, and I often send people away with a few remedies to have on hand in an attempt to anticipate what is required).*

30.4.08 Sam had one dose of (5) Lach 200, without any obvious aggravation or improvement, then he took one dose of (4) DPT M which seemed to help overall, but his face became puffy, and moods fluctuated.
8.5.08 Is more settled.
16.7.08 He is improving really well. Lots of people have commented on how much better he is. Repeat (4) DPT M.
Rx. (6) DPT 10M (not to take until advised).

5.8.08 (5th consultation). Has given the 6 doses of (5).
Two weeks ago, got a cold with ear pin then hot and cold sweats followed by a sore throat. Was helped with Belladonna 6.
NOW: has massive night sweats without fever. Is easily fatigued. Responds emotionally. Climbs a lot.
Digestive problems are still an issue with burping and chest pains, possibly worse following the homoeopathic remedies.

His behaviour is really good. The anxiety and hyperactivity are significantly less. No meltdowns anymore – the teachers say that Sam is now better behaved than other children in his class.
His language skills are improving, and he is catching up with others.
Rx. (6) DPT 10M (use this now), hold (7) Hepatitis B M (use if still burping).

22.9.08 Sam started banging his head and screaming at night (an old symptom returning). Digestive symptoms are still an issue.
Rx. Give 1 dose of (7).
21.10.08 Language is still improving, but he has been socially upset lately. His stools changed after (6).
Rx. Advised to give one dose of (1) MMR M, (4) DPT M, (7) Hep B M with one week between each dose. Repeat as appropriate.
22.12.08 After (4) DPT M had 4-5 huge bowel movements a day for 4 days, plus mucus around the stool. The less hyperactive, but still aggressive. Puffy eyes.
Rx. Advised to wait until mid-January 2009 then repeat (6) DPT 10M
24.3.09 A week after the dose of (6) began stuttering and eyes twitched. Yelling. Now is at kinder crying and tired. The doctor said Sam's iron levels were low.
Rx 1 dose of (1) MMR M. Femax (a herbal iron supplement).

12.5.09 (6th consultation). Gut problems. Low iron levels. Doctor gave cod liver oil and iron supplements, which made Sam very agitated.

After his reaction to the (6) on 24.3.09 saw another practitioner who gave Sam CALC c 30 AT NIGHT. Relived some coughing and nightly sweats, but gave him nightmares.
At kinder the teacher says Sam is very bright, but his anxiety holds him back, especially anxiety about what to do next.
He is a perfectionist, can be obsessive. Wants to control his own situation (not others). He knows when he fails, and this is difficult for him at the moment. There is a strong family history of anxiety.
Very good now with counting (mental development continuing)
He shows off. Cries a lot. But is friendly with everyone, although sometimes something triggers a reaction.
If the sun is out he wants to play outside. But he is heat sensitive.
Alternating constipation and diarrhoea. Very hungry. His cravings have changed – he now hates milk and eggs, and likes salty and spicy foods.
NEW SYMPTOM> Fear of the dark. Wants to know where his mother is. Refuses to go to bed, and when he does needs a light on in his room.
Parents removed Sam from the early intervention program which they felt was too confrontational.
Rx. (7) Arg Nit 30, and (8) Arg Nit 200 to hold. (Note: used the number (7) twice)

9.6.09 Initially aggravated on (7). Now needs to give it weekly, and it is helping Sam.

16.9.09 (7th consultation). Sam is going really well in general. The (7) and (8) helped him a lot (mother said that every remedy does one thing, removes a problem, then he changes). Not so worried about the dark, and hyperactivity has changed a lot. No longer anxious at kinder about new activities. Is very compliant with very few tears now. Socially is much better.
DIAGNOSIS FROM DOCTOR: Sam is no longer autistic, and is now ADHD – now diagnosed as having APD (auditory processing disorder),

i.e. he can hear information but cannot process it – he is overloaded because he has acute hearing. CNS causing this. Sam did very well on cognitive tests, but verbal IQ was low. Can have trouble too much information (will jump up and down on the spot).
Dr recommended speech therapy and visual learning aids at school.

Now, especially if he is tired, he will nag a bit. Gut issues are better since removing dairy foods.
He had a croup infection on an off for 2 months - plus a 24 hour rash in the middle of this (helped with Pulsatilla).
Salt and spicy cravings gone. Wants bread now. Eats very quickly. If he eats regularly his moods are better.
Rx. (6) DPT 10M – give Sam 1 sniff of the remedy. Use (7) and (8) Arg Nit if needed emotionally. (9) Hypericum 30 daily dose (to support CNS).

10.5.10 (8th consultation). (*Note – no communication for 8 months*).
In November 2009 was diagnosed with whooping cough – not confirmed with swabs. Saw a local practitioner, and it took some time to settle. (*Note – Sam had been taking occasional doses of DPT 10M, and it is uncertain whether he had the disease, or a very deep clearing reaction to the vaccine, especially the Pertussis (whooping cough) component*).
Still has a cough that comes and goes.
No more symptoms of autism, ADHD, or a learning disability. At school is doing very well. Sam's language is now in the normal range (*remember that Sam's parents originally were told he would not be able to attend normal school*).
Last week had vomiting and diarrhoea (reaction to food or old symptoms? – last had this following MMR vaccine).

OVERVIEW: Sam has passed through a period of significant physical "sickness" (which may or may not have been a final clearing reaction), and now is very much better.

A new program of treatment was now started looking at remaining issues which are clearly more "normal" in the sense of being typical constitutional issues faced by many children. It would appear that the vaccine layers have been substantially or fully removed. However, IF symptoms suggest an occasional dose of high potency DPT or MMR remedies, they will be used.
For the practitioner, this type of result is what we work for – a fundamental change in the wellbeing of a seriously unwell person. It provides more satisfaction than mere $$ alone could supply.

1.8 Case 18 - "Jim"

Overview: Jim's case is different from most others because at the time I did not have a potency of the Hepatitis B vaccine, a clear "never well since" trigger, but I did have the Hepatitis B nosode. This remedy appeared to have a positive effect, despite not covering the chemicals in the vaccine itself. The next remedy, a potency of the DPT vaccine, appeared to take up the case and progress it.

I saw Jim on 1st June, 2001. He was nearly 15 years old, in Year 9 at school. His mother said he was continually sick.

He currently suffered from sore dry throats, swollen glands, blocked ears, recurring colds, his bones ached, and he was often tired and cranky. His tonsils were enlarged, and the lining of his nose is swollen, although a sinus scan was clear. Blood tests showed nothing.

He was never well since a series of three Hepatitis B vaccines on 24/2/99, 31/3/99, and 15/9/99. He was ill with a cough on 16/10/99 and again on 10/11/99 and has been generally unwell since then.

He had a severe 24-hour reaction to his first DPT vaccine. After that he was given each component separately. He had ear infections when young.

Rx. (1) Hepatitis B M, single dose. (2) Phytolacca 6c, 2 pillules twice daily *(note: the Phytolaca 6 was used as a lymphatic drainage remedy)*

27.7.01 (2nd consultation)
Fewer headaches. Better in the morning, but still tired during the day. Still has phlegm. Lately, sleep poor. However, in general feeling better.

Rx. Sinus herbal drops. (3) Hepatitis B 10M every three weeks.

28.8.01. Mother phoned. He is still improving, although still is congested.

4.12.01 (3rd consultation)
Very few headaches now. All the Hep B related symptoms have cleared (sore throats etc).
Recently, his stomach has been uncomfortable.

Rx. (4) DPT 10M every 2 weeks. Sinus herbal drops. Kali Sulph 6x t.d.s. *(note: these last two remedies were used as drainage to assist with acutely clearing the sinuses when necessary).*

17.2.02 Phoned. Going very well
x. (5) DPT 50M every 3 weeks.
CASE FINISHED

Question 2: What are the Symptoms of Vaccine Injury?

2.1 Symptoms of Vaccines Injury

Orthodox medical journals report details of many adverse events arising from vaccination, as do the handbooks produced by Health Departments in most developed countries and even vaccine inserts supplied by manufacturers.

Yet the same authors claim that vaccination is basically safe, and certainly much less dangerous than the possible adverse effects of the diseases which the vaccines are aimed to prevent, thus making vaccination acceptable.

As noted earlier, researchers have not reported in orthodox medical journals comprehensive research into the long-term impact of vaccines on the general wellbeing of recipients. **So, any statement that vaccines are less damaging than the diseases they are designed to prevent cannot be "scientific".** This is a major point which has not been taken up within orthodox medicine or health bureaucracies.

In our attempt to quantify the adverse effects of vaccines, it is helpful to separate symptoms of vaccine injury into short-term reactions and long-term injury.

2.2 Short-Term Reactions

Any Health Department handbook on vaccines will list possible short-term reactions to vaccines. For example, the list produced by the South Australian Health Department is typical. Table 4 presents an example of common adverse events following vaccination was publicly released by the South Australian Government Ref: http://www.dh.sa.gov.au/pehs/Immunisation/adverse-events-vaccines.pdf.

That reference is no longer available, but a very similar list is shown at

https://immunisationhandbook.health.gov.au/resources/handbook-tables/table-common-side-effects-following-immunisation-for-vaccines-used-in-the-national-immunisation-program-schedule (accessed 31/8/2023).

Table 4: Adverse Events Following Vaccination

Vaccine	Side effects of vaccination
DTPa Diphtheria Tetanus Pertussis (acellular)	DTPa vaccine (Serious adverse events are less common than with DTPw) *Irritable, crying, unsettled and generally unhappy Drowsiness or tiredness *Localized pain, redness & swelling at injection site *Occasionally injection site nodule. may last many weeks (no treatment needed) *Low grade temperature (fever)
Hepatitis B	*Localized pain, redness & swelling at injection site *Occasionally injection site nodule. may last many weeks (no treatment needed) *Low grade temperature (fever)
Hib	*Localized pain, redness & swelling at injection site *Occasionally injection site nodule. may last many weeks (no treatment needed) *Low grade temperature (fever)
Influenza	*Drowsiness or tiredness *Muscle aches *Localized pain, redness & swelling at injection site *Occasionally injection site nodule. may last many weeks (no treatment needed) *Low grade temperature (fever)
MMR Measles	*Occasionally injection site nodule. may last many weeks (no treatment needed) *Seen 7 to 10 days after vaccination:

Vaccine	Side effects of vaccination
Mumps Rubella	*Low grade temperature (fever) lasting 2-3 days, faint red rash (not infectious), head cold and/or runny nose, cough and/or puffy eyes *Drowsiness or tiredness S welling of salivary glands
Meningococcal type C	*Irritable, crying, unsettled and generally unhappy *Loss of appetite *Headache (usually observed in adolescent/adults) *Localized pain, redness & swelling at injection site *Occasionally injection site nodule. may last many weeks (no treatment needed) *Low grade temperature (fever)
Pneumococcal (7vPCV) (23vPPV)	Conjugate vaccine (7vPCV) *Localized pain, redness & swelling at injection site *Occasionally injection site nodule. may last many weeks (no treatment needed) *Low grade temperature (fever) Polysaccharide vaccine (23vPPV) *Localized pain, redness & swelling at injection site *Occasionally injection site nodule. may last many weeks (no treatment needed) *Low grade temperature (fever)
Polio	OPV: (Oral Polio Vaccine) *Occasional diarrhoea (no treatment usually needed but parent or carer must wash hands carefully after changing nappies) IPV: (Inactivated Polio Vaccine – injected) *Muscle aches *Localized pain, redness & swelling at injection site *Occasionally injection site nodule. may last many weeks (no treatment needed) *Low grade temperature (fever)
Rubella	*Bruising or bleeding *Local inflammation and discomfort *Swollen glands *Localized pain, stiff neck, joint pains *Rash *Low grade temperature (fever)
Varicella	*Localized pain, redness & swelling at injection site *Occasionally injection site nodule. may last many weeks (no

Vaccine	Side effects of vaccination
(chickenpox)	treatment needed) *Low grade temperature (fever) *Seen 5-26 days after vaccination: *Pustular rash (2-5 lesions) usually at injection site which occasional covers other parts of the body

If the above list represented the only ill-effects of vaccines, and their duration was brief, then many would accept them without concern. Others would still point to the immediate potential dangers of death and permanent brain injury. These happen very rarely, and this low incidence is accepted by the pharmaceutical industry, although not by many parents.

2.2.1 The VAERS Database

Another source of information regarding mainly short-term effects, although death and brain injury are included, is the US Governments ***Vaccine Adverse Events Reporting Service*** (VAERS), available at https://vaers.hhs.gov/ (accessed 10/6/23).

The VAERS website (15/2/2019) stated: "Established in 1990, the Vaccine Adverse Event Reporting System (VAERS) is a national early warning system to detect possible safety problems in U.S.-licensed vaccines. VAERS is co-managed by the Centres for Disease Control and Prevention (CDC) and the U.S. Food and Drug Administration (FDA). VAERS accepts and analyses reports of adverse events (possible side effects) after a person has received a vaccination. Anyone can report an adverse event to VAERS. Healthcare professionals are required to report certain adverse events and vaccine manufacturers are required to report all adverse events that come to their attention.

VAERS is a passive reporting system, meaning it relies on individuals to send in reports of their experiences to CDC and FDA. VAERS is not designed to determine if a vaccine caused a health problem, but is especially useful for detecting unusual or unexpected patterns of adverse event reporting that might indicate a possible safety problem with a vaccine. This way, VAERS can provide CDC and FDA with valuable information that additional work and evaluation is necessary to further assess a possible safety concern."

VAERS provide massive data sets of vaccine injury which anyone can access at https://vaers.hhs.gov/data.html or https://vaers.hhs.gov/data/datasets.html (accessed 10/6/23). Vaccine advocates warn that this information is misleading because it comes mainly from parents of vaccine injured children, but it shows the "tip of the iceberg" of vaccine injury as it is agreed that most events remain unreported – see Rosenthal S & Chen R. The reporting sensitivities of two passive surveillance systems for vaccine adverse events. *Am J Public Health.* 1995 December; 85(12): 1706–1709 (accessed 31/8/23).

2.2.2 Vaccine Inserts

As mentioned in Section 1, vaccine inserts provide information about vaccine reactions and injury, both short and long term, but mainly listing immediate reactions observed in short-term trials.

But the real problem with vaccination relates to the long-term adverse reactions which are rarely acknowledged in the orthodox literature.

2.3 Long-term Injury

There are two ways to measure long-term vaccine injury, and we shall consider them in turn.

2.3(a) Predicted and observed vaccine effects: Vaxxed V's Unvaxxed Children

Orthodox claims concerning the long-term safety of vaccines are unscientific for one very simple reason; the orthodox community has published no significant research of the long-term impact of vaccination on the total wellbeing of recipients, thus making impossible a "scientific" comparison between the risks from diseases and the full risks from vaccination.

One exception is the research by Dr Michel Odent, and it was arrived at by accident. In 1994, Dr Odent reported the results of his study of the effects of breast feeding on the long-term wellbeing of children in the orthodox journals the *Lancet*, the *British Medical Journal* and *JAMA*. He expected to find that the fully breastfed children in his study would be generally healthier than the non-breastfed children. He used the incidence of asthma, eczema, ear/hearing problems, and hospitalisation experience to indicate general wellness. To his surprise he found that within the breastfed group there was a relatively healthy group, and a relatively unhealthy group.

Odent determined that the factor separating these two groups of breastfed children was vaccination. His data showed that children who received the pertussis vaccine were 5.43 times more likely to develop asthma in later years, over twice as likely to have ear infections, and significantly more likely to spend longer periods in hospital than those who had not received the vaccine.

[Odent M et al, Atopic Eczema. *Lancet*. 1994: 344; p.140.
Odent M, Culpin EE, Kimmel T. Pertussis vaccination and asthma: Is there a link? *JAMA*. 1994: 272(8); pp.592-3.

Odent M et al, (1994c) Pertussis Vaccination and Asthma: Is There a Link? *British Medical Journal*, Vol 272; pp. 592-3].

It is likely that if Odent reported his work today he would be attacked by the medical establishment. In fact, it is probable that the three journals would not publish his findings today.

Other articles have indirectly supported Odent's hypothesis regarding a link between asthma and DPT vaccination. For example, Kemp and colleagues studied 1,265 children in Christchurch, New Zealand, born in 1977. The 23 who were not vaccinated against DPT and Polio had no recorded asthma or other allergic illnesses before the age of 10. In the immunised children, 23.1% had asthma, 22.5% had asthma consultations, and 30.0% had consultations for other allergic illnesses. Similar differences were observed at ages 5 and 16 years.
[Kemp T et al, (1997). Is infant immunization a risk factor for childhood asthma or allergy? *Epidemiology*. Nov; 8(6); pp. 678-80.]

A study in 2007 by Nakajima and colleagues using data from the Tasmanian Asthma Study, examined the link between vaccination and atopic diseases in a group of Tasmanians born in 1961, and who were followed in 1968, 1974, and 1991. The authors claimed that their study "seems to be the first prospective cohort study examining the association between multiple immunizations in childhood and atopic outcomes up to the age of 30 years".
The authors concluded that "our study provides evidence that some immunization may be associated with a small increased risk of atopic disease, mostly eczema by age 7 years; the evidence for an association with asthma risk was minimal".
[Nakajima K et at (2007) Is childhood immunization associated with atopic disease from age 7 to 32 years? *Thorax*, 62:270-275,]

However, their data provides for a different interpretation. Table 5 below shows **only data which is statistically significant** (P<0.05) from their Table 3, *Association between immunization and childhood atopic* *diseases: ORs adjusted for sex, birthplace, history of bacterial infection, parental smoking, parental asthma, history of viral infection, birth order and history of pneumonia.*

In every case, children vaccinated with the nominated vaccine are more likely to have the condition identified than non-vaccinated children (this is shown when the Odds Ratio (OR) is greater than 1).

Table 5: Statistically significant outcomes from Nakajima et al Table 3

Outcome	Vaccine	OR (95% CI)	P Value
Asthma by age 7	Diphtheria	1.33 (1.06 to 1.68)	0.01
Eczema by age 7 years	Diphtheria	1.53 (1.13 to 2.07)	<0.01
	Tetanus	1.53 (1.15 to 2.04)	<0.01
	Pertussis	1.46 (1.10 to 1.87)	< 0.01
	Polio	1.36 (1.00 to 1.87)	0.05
Food allergy by age 7 yrs	Diphtheria	1.47 (1.04 to 2.07)	0.03
	Pertussis	1.39 (1.01 to 1.91)	0.04
	Polio	1.44 (1.00 to 2.07)	0.05

I extended Odent's work in my doctoral studies in 2004. I examined four groups of children aged between 4 and 12 years of age, including vaccinated children, those who used HP, those who used general/constitutional prevention, and those who used no method of immunisation.

To measure overall wellbeing, I examined the incidence of asthma, eczema, ear/hearing problems, allergies and behavioural problems. I also tested whether the conditions were diagnosed by a GP, or not. The resulting 40 possible outcomes were compared using odd ratios and Chi Squared probability tests. The results for the vaccinated and HP groups are shown in Table 6.

[Golden I (2005) *The Potential Value of Homœoprophylaxis in the Prevention of Infectious Diseases, and the maintenance of General Health in Recipients* Swinburne University Press, Melbourne.]

The **figures in bold type are statistically significant (P<0.05).** An Odds Ratio >1 indicates a positive association between the condition and the immunisation option. If the Odds Ratio is <1, the immunisation method is associated with a reduced incidence of the condition. The **P** reading indicates the likelihood of the results being coincidental. So **P** = 0.05 represents a 95% level of confidence in the results.

Table 6 Comparative Safety of Vaccination and Homœoprophylaxis

		All Diagnoses		**GP Diagnoses**	
Condition	**Measurement**	**HP only**	**Vacc'n only**	**HP only**	**Vacc'n only**
Asthma	Odds Ratio	**0.117**	**1.75**	**0.124**	**1.89**
	Chi Test P	**0.0004**	**0.0025**	**0.0006**	**0.0007**
Eczema	Odds Ratio	**0.382**	1.315	**0.239**	**1.76**
	Chi Test P	**0.0146**	0.121	**0.0097**	**0.006**
Ear/ Hearing	Odds Ratio	0.917	1.149	0.703	**1.517**
	Chi Test P	0.792	0.459	0.364	**0.04**
Allergies	Odds Ratio	0.550	1.220	**0.307**	1.518
	Chi Test P	0.074	0.239	**0.038**	0.061
Behaviour	Odds Ratio	0.446	0.869	**0.541**	0.784
	Chi Test P	0.170	0.593	**0.055**	0.613

[Golden I. Homoeoprophylaxis: A Fifteen Year Clinical Study. Isaac Golden Publications. Gisborne, Victoria. 2004].

Ideally, we want the Odds Ratio to be very close to zero with **P** less than 0.05. When the Odds Ratio is greater than 1, this means the method is probably one of the triggering causes of the condition.

For all conditions where the results were statistically significant, vaccination was associated with an increased incidence of the condition, and HP with a reduced incidence of the condition. **The figures showed that vaccinated children are 15 times more likely to have asthma than children using HP**, and 7 times more likely to have skin problems. They are likely to have higher levels of ear/hearing problems, allergies and behavioural problems, but the latter comparisons were not all statistically significant. Vaccinated children were also significantly less healthy than both the general/constitutional group, and the group that used no method of immunisation.

Since that time, other studies have examined the relationship between vaccination and the incidence chronic disease.

Generation Rescue. (2007) *Cal-Oregan vaccinated v's unvaccinated survey.* http://www.rense.com/general78/unvac.htm (accessed 1/6/19)

Generation Rescue, an autism support group, commissioned an independent opinion research firm, *SurveyUSA* of Verona NJ, to conduct a telephone survey in nine counties in California and Oregon. Counties were selected by Generation Rescue. Interviews were successfully completed in 11,817 households with one or more children aged 4 to 17. From those 11,817 households, data on 17,674 children was gathered. Of the 17,674 children inventoried, 991 were described as completely unvaccinated. For each unvaccinated child, a health battery was administered[17].

Generation Rescue chose to use telephone interviews with parents to gather data on children so as to closely mirror the methodology the

Centre for Disease Control (CDC) uses to establish national prevalence for neurological disorders (ND) such as ADHD and autism through their national phone survey of parent responses. Generation Rescue chose to focus on children ages 4-17 to match the age range used by CDC. The data for boys is shown in Table 3 (boys comprised roughly 80% of ND cases).

Table 3: The Generation Rescue Results - Boys

BOYS	UV = Un Vacc.		PV = Parti'ly Vacc.		FV = Fully Vacc.		AV = All Vacc.		Ratio FV/ UV
	#	%	#	%	#	%	#	%	
Number of children	**533**	**100**	**906**	**100**	**7736**	**100**	**8642**	**100**	
Number with any diagnosis	53	10	225	25	2026	26	2251	26	2.6
Number with ASD (any one of c,d,e)	21	4	76	8	357	5	433	5	1.3
Number with ASD or AD (any one of a-e)	29	5	141	16	1060	14	1201	14	2.6
Number with ADD	13	2	69	8	586	8	655	8	3.1
Number with ADHD	12	2	56	6	575	7	631	7	3.2
Number with Asperger's	10	2	31	3	184	2	215	2	1.3

Number with PDD-NOS	7	1	22	2	82	1	104	1	0.9
Number with Austism	12	2	61	7	253	3	314	4	1.6
Number with Asthma	36	7	122	13	1246	16	1368	16	2.3
Number with Juvenile Diabetes	11	2	7	1	48	1	55	1	0.3
Condit'ns	**204**	**38**	**810**	**89**	**6,417**	**83**	**7,227**	**84**	**2.2**

Bachmair A (2012) State of health of unvaccinated children. www.vaccineinjury.info/ (accessed 16/7/19).

Bachmair has to date collected health data on 10,468 unvaccinated children using a question-set partially similar to the KiGGS study noted in the Introduction. He also collected additional information and used other published studies for conditions which were not covered by KiGGS[18]. This allowed a comparison between a comparable number of vaccinated and unvaccinated children (rather than a mere 94 in KiGGS). The information was contributed by parents and lacks the random selection of the KiGGS study and therefore may contain unreliable data. However what Bachmair's study lacks in rigour it makes up in both relevance and volume of data. Once again, a comparison of the KiGGS and other data with the Bachmair data reveals clear differences between vaccinated and unvaccinated children, the latter being in general healthier than their vaccinated peers. These findings are summarised in Table 4. It should be noted that Bachmair's ratios will probably understate the differences due to the limitations of the KiGGS study noted earlier (not filtering out age-inappropriate or partially vaccinated children).

Table 4: Likelihood of condition in vaccinated (KiGGS and other) children compared to unvaccinated (Bachmair) children

Condition	Ratio
Asthma	1.9
Eczema	1.8
Ear/Hearing	1.6
Allergies	2.1
ADHD	4.0
Hayfever	3.6
Sinusitis	13.3
Epilepsy	9

Mawson AR, Ray BD, Bhuiyan AR, Jacob B. Pilot comparative study on the health of vaccinated and unvaccinated 6- to 12-year-old U.S. children *J Transl Sci,* 2017: 3(3) ; 12-12. 2017 doi: 10.15761/JTS.1000186 (accessed 17.7.19).

This study aimed 1) to compare vaccinated and unvaccinated children on a broad range of health outcomes, and 2) to determine whether an association found between vaccination and neurodevelopmental disorders (NDD), if any, remained significant after adjustment for other measured factors.

A cross-sectional study of mothers of children educated at home was carried out in collaboration with home-school organizations in four U.S. states: Florida, Louisiana, Mississippi and Oregon. Mothers were asked to complete an anonymous online questionnaire on their 6- to 12-year-old biological children with respect to pregnancy-related factors, birth history, vaccinations, physician diagnosed illnesses, medications used, and health services. NDD, a derived diagnostic measure, was defined as having one or more of the following three closely related diagnoses: a learning disability, Attention Deficient Hyperactivity Disorder, and Autism Spectrum Disorder.

A convenience sample of 666 children was obtained, of which 261 (39%) were unvaccinated. The vaccinated were less likely than the unvaccinated to have been diagnosed with chickenpox and pertussis, but more likely to have been diagnosed with pneumonia, otitis media, allergies and NDD. After adjustment, vaccination, male gender, and preterm birth remained significantly associated with NDD. However, in a final adjusted model with interaction, vaccination but not preterm birth remained associated with NDD, while the interaction of preterm birth and vaccination was associated with 6.6-fold increased odds of NDD (95% CI: 2.8, 15.5).

In conclusion, vaccinated home-school children were found to have a higher rate of allergies and NDD than unvaccinated home-school children.

Morgensen SW, Anderson A, Rodrigues A, Benn CS, Aaby P. The Introduction of Diphtheria-Tetanus-Pertussis and Oral Polio vaccine Among Young Infants in an Urban African Community: A Natural Experiment. *EBioMedicine.* 2017: 17;192-198. http://dx.doi.org/10.1016/j.ebiom.2017.01.041 (accessed 17.7.19).

The authors examined the introduction of diphtheria-tetanus-pertussis (DTP) and oral polio vaccine (OPV) in an urban community in Guinea-Bissau in the early 1980s. The child population had been followed with 3-monthly nutritional weighing sessions since 1978. From June 1981 DTP and OPV were offered from 3 months of age at these sessions. Due to the 3-monthly intervals between sessions, the children were allocated by birthday in a 'natural experiment' to receive vaccinations early or late between 3 and 5 months of age. We included children who were <6 months of age when vaccinations started and children born until the end of December 1983. We compared mortality between 3 and 5 months of age of DTP-vaccinated and not-yet-DTP-vaccinated children in Cox proportional hazard models.

Among 3-5-month-old children, having received DTP (±OPV) was associated with a mortality hazard ratio (HR) of 5.00 (95% CI 1.53-16.3) compared with not-yet-DTP-vaccinated children. Differences in background factors did not explain the effect. The negative effect was particularly strong for children who had received DTP-only and no OPV (HR=10.0 (2.61-38.6)). All-cause infant mortality after 3months of age increased after the introduction of these vaccines (HR=2.12 (1.07-4.19)). The authors concluded that DTP was associated with increased mortality; OPV may modify the effect of DTP.

Summary of Studies

Table 7 is presented in two parts due to its size. It summarises the findings of the seven studies discussed above. The numbers greater than 1 show the number of times the condition being studied is MORE likely to be present in vaccinated children compared with completely unvaccinated children. **If the number is less than 1 it means the condition is LESS likely in vaccinated compared with unvaccinated children.**

None of the numbers are less than 1.

Table 7: Likelihood of condition in vaccinated compared to unvaccinated children

Condition	Odent (446)	Golden (645)		
		HP only	General only	Nothing
Asthma	**5.43**	**15.2**	3.9	**2.7**
Eczema	1.28	**7.4**	**7.8**	**2.6**
Ear/Hearing	**1.89**	2.2	2.5	**3.8**
Allergies	-	**4.9**	3.4	**2.5**
Behaviour (general)	-	1.5	2.1	1.0
ADHD	-	-	-	-
Autism	-	-	-	-
Epilepsy	-	-	-	-
Hayfever	-	-	-	-
Sinusitis	-	-	-	-
All/other conditions	1.44	**2.7**	9.4	**2.1**
Death (DTP)				

Table 7: (cont)

Condition	Gen. Res. (boys) (9,175)	Nakajima	Bachmair Vs KiGGS (23,845)	Mawson (666)	Morgensen (1,057)
Asthma	2.3	**1.33**	1.9		
Eczema	-	**1.5**	1.8	**2.9**	
Ear/Hearing	-		1.6	**3.8**	
Allergies	-	**1.4**	2.1	**3.9**	
Behaviour (general)	-		-	**3.7**	
ADHD	3.2		4.0	**4.2**	
Autism	1.6		-	**4.2**	
Epilepsy	-		9.0		

Hayfever	-		3.6	**30.1**	
Sinusitis	-		13.3		
All/other conditions	2.6		-	**2.4**	
Death (DTP)					**5.0**

I published an article in 2019 which included a summary of these studies.
Golden I. Reluctance to vaccinate: Reasons and solutions. *Journal of Translational Science*. **2019**. Vol 5: 2-6 doi: 10.15761/JTS.1000326

In that article I calculated (i) a simple average of results, (ii) a weighted average of results, and (iii) a simple average of statistically significant results for each condition. These figures are indicative only and are re-presented in Table 8 following. **However, they clearly indicate that the case for undertaking a substantial analysis of long-term vaccine effects is overwhelming.**

Some pro-pharmaceutical authors claim that a substantial study to confirm the long-term effects of vaccination would be unethical because it would deny children protection. Such claims are rubbish, as the study needed is a retrospective one and the decision whether or not to vaccinate would have been made by parents years before the analysis.

Some claim the study is not needed and that there already is plenty of evidence that vaccines are safe. Yet the attempt to prevent confirmation of whether these preliminary findings can be replicated on a larger scale can have only one goal – to deny parents and politicians access to the truth. If large-scale studies proved that there was definitely no link between vaccination and chronic illness, then it would change the views of many vaccine hesitators. If it proved there was a link, then politicians would be forced to make different choices.

Table 8: Likelihood of condition in vaccinated compared to unvaccinated children (indicative average measures)

Condition	Simple Average	Weighted Average	Simple Average of Statistically Significant Figures
Asthma	4.7	2.4	6.2
Eczema	3.6	2.4	4.4
Ear/Hearing	2.6	1.7	3.2
Allergies	3.0	2.0	12.7
Behaviour (general)	2.1	3.0	3.7
ADHD	3.8	3.8	4.2
Autism	2.9	1.8	4.2
Epilepsy	9.0	9.0	-
Hayfever	16.9	4.3	30.1
Sinusitis	13.3	13.3	-
All/other conditions	3.4	2.3	2.4
Learning Disabilities	5.2	5.2	5.2

NOTE: The numbers indicate how many times more likely it is that the vaccinated child will have the condition than the unvaccinated child.

So predicted and observed long-term effects suggest that vaccines are one cause of long-term diseases in recipients.

It is to the discredit of drug companies that they have not researched the long-term impact of vaccination on overall wellbeing (or if they have, they have not published the data). It is to the discredit of Health

Departments and politicians that they have not insisted that such research be undertaken before forcing vaccines on many children.

The Kennedy-Hooker Evidence

I literally just received my copy of the book ***Vax-Unvax: Let the Science Speak*** by Robert F Kennedy Jr and Dr Brian Hooker (6th September 2023). It is a significant contribution to the evidence base, and rather than lift some studies from the book and insert them into the preceding Tables which I presented in earlier editions of this book, I would recommend that those readers who want to add considerably to their knowledge about the differences in the health of vaccinated and unvaccinated children obtain their own copy of their impressive book.

I was disappointed that they did not acknowledge the pioneering work by Dr Michel Odent. Given they cited articles from the *Journal of Translational Science* they should have seen my 2019 article cited above which referred to Dr Odent's work. But that is a small failure given the value of their contribution.

Their work demonstrates, yet again, that the leaders of pharmaceutical medicine intentionally refuse to undertake needed studies comparing the long-term health of vaccinated and unvaccinated children for one simple reason – they know that objective evidence will demonstrate that vaccines cause chronic illness, and that those few who financially benefit from the suffering of many remain unaccountable, and that if parents knew the truth they would be disgusted, and angry, and demand change.

2.3(b) Evaluation of conditions resolved by treatment

Another way to assess possible long-term vaccine injury is to come at the problem backwards, i.e., tabulate the health conditions suspected to be caused by vaccination which have responded to specific vaccine-injury treatment. For example, if a patient whose asthma is suspected as being triggered by the DPT vaccine is given homeopathic potencies of the vaccine, **and** the asthma improves for no other apparent reason, then **we can conclude with a high level of confidence that the DPT vaccine caused the asthma because the DPT potencies will generally ONLY work if the vaccine is the cause.**

Pioneering work in this area was also been reported by the late Dr Tinus Smits. See http://www.tinussmits.com/3734/home.aspx (accessed 31/8/2023).

Working independently, we came to remarkably similar conclusions regarding the probable long-term health effects of vaccination based on our results from treating vaccine injured children over 20 years. Table 9 summarises a comparison I made in 2001 of some of our results for 52 children (26 each) with 100 presenting conditions.

Asthma and respiratory conditions were significant, as were skin problems. Conditions relating to mental/emotional/nervous system problems were also very significant. This is consistent with the work by Odent, Kemp, Nakajima and I reported above.

More of Dr Smits work is shown in Appendix 3.

Remember that the percentage figures are very similar even though at that time Dr Smits and I had never communicated and were not aware of each other's work. A great validation of the figures.

Table 9 Conditions Responding to Treatment for Vaccine Injury

	Golden		Smits		Total	
	#	%	#	%	#	%
Behavioural problems; Speech/learning problems; Autism; Epilepsy; Tourette's syndrome; Listlessness; Sleep disturbance	16	32.7	17	33.3	33	33.0
Upper respiratory tract problems; Ears/hearing problems; Asthma; Lower respiratory tract problems	20	40.8	18	35.3	38	38.0
Skin problems	6	12.2	8	15.7	14	14.0
Allergies Gastrointestinal problems Raynaud's; Arthritis; Migraines	2 2 3	4.1 4.1 6.1	1 7 0	2.0 13.7 0.0	393	3.0 9.0 3.0
TOTALS	**49**	**100.0**	**51**	**100.0**	**100**	**100.0**

The above studies, whilst of use, do not separate vaccine injury by individual vaccines.

The Tables and Figures in Section 2.6 following show my latest research data on the treatment of vaccine injured children classified according to vaccines treated.

*This material is based on a study of **818** case files where potencies of the relevant vaccines were used to treat suspected cases of vaccine injury. Of the 818 cases, there was no follow up in 184 cases. In the remaining 634 there were positive results in 429 cases (and 43 cases where there was no improvement or the patient was worse, and 162 still to be decided).*
The conditions treated in these successful cases, as well as in all cases, are examined in detail.

But before then we shall look at two cases:

2.4 Case 504 – "Geraldine"

Overview: This is a simple case which is included because despite being diagnosed as being on the Autism Spectrum the first and only remedy used was DPT HEXA in several potencies.
There was no direct clue as to which dose of vaccine lead to problems, and the key symptom that concerned parents was her severe meltdowns which fitted the DPT picture better than MMR. This is where the summaries of common vaccine symptoms can be of use when selecting a remedy.

23.11.18. 1st consultation. Female. 31 months.

Vaccinated 2, 4, 6, 12, 18 months. No obvious reactions.

Has been diagnosed on the Spectrum.

Late with her milestones: crawled – 13 months; walked 19 months; words – none,
No interaction with other children.

Very sensitive to noise (e.g. vacuum cleaner).

Good pregnancy. Caesarean.

Colic? With minimal sleep. 4 months settled, slept through by 8 months.
Did not feed well – had breast milk and formula (wouldn't feed well).
NAN – projectile vomiting. 2 weeks Carrie care and the vomiting stopped.

NOW: Is a great eater and sleeper.

Loves books. Loves drawing (fine motor skills are OK). Loves stickers. Loves her bedroom.

Understands and is normally compliant.

NOW: every couple of days she can have meltdowns if she doesn't get her own way.
Worse 3-4 pm, or strange places.
Hand flapping a lot. Is usually happy.
Trembles at times.
Very occasional toes walking.
Lots of cuddles with mum (but she won't initiate it).

Rx. (1) DPT 30 – 1 pill x 2 weekly. Then (2) DPT 200 – 1 pill x 2 weekly.

28.11.15. Better eye contact. No tantrums. Is a bit more unsettled at night before bed.

17.1.19 Has settled on (1). Possibly aggravated on (2).

29.3.19 Is much better. Saying more words, and is more calm.

Rx. (3) DPT M – 1 pill weekly for 3 doses, Then (4) DPT 10M – 1 pill weekly for 3 doses.

10.5.19 Is going well.

Rx. (5) DPT 50M. 1 pill every 10 days.

NOTE: This case is not finished, and it is likely that once the vaccine layer(s) have been cleared a constitutional remedy will finish the case. However, the DPT HEXA remedy has made a significant difference to Geraldine in just 6 months.

2.5 Case 418 - "Ned"

In this case potencies of MMR were used in conjunction with the brain powder formulated by Dr Smits. Ned made good progress over 19 months. I then heard from the parents that due to legal changes affecting pre-school entry in Victoria, Australia, they had decided to vaccinate their children, and I did not hear from them again. I don't know if Ned regressed or not.

11.3.2013. 1st consultation.

25 mths old. Vaccinated at 2, 4, 6, 12, and 18 months.

At around 18 months a health nurse told parents that Ned had poor eye contact (this is better now).

He had simple words at around 9 months – "mumma" and "dada" - they were lost. Has no language now.
Was experimenting with different foods at 12 months. Then around 13 months had gastro and stopped eating well. Now is very selective with food. Will have wheatbix, toasted sandwich (jam/ pb/cheese), 2-minute noodles and cheese. Maybe a hot dog. Biscuits at night.

Now, tries to initiate contact with other children but doesn't succeed, possibly because he has no language.
Other development seems good physically. Hearing is OK.

Rx. (1) MMR30 x 2 weekly for 2 weeks then (2) MMR 200 x 2 weekly then report.

18.3.13 After (1) he showed an increase in affection, eye contact is better. He is stumbling more. Possible bad dreams.

28.3.13 Better at crèche. Eye contact is improving. Rx. (3) MMR M x2 weekly and (4) MMR 10M x2 weekly. Nutritional compound.
7.4.13 Diarrhoea. Stop compound and slowly build up.

13.5.13 2nd consultation.

Nutritional powder gave diarrhoea.
Has given (4) x 2 weekly in water for 2 weeks.

Has definitely progressed over the last 2 months.
More affectionate with family – is kissing his parents now.
Jigsaw puzzles – he can recognise animals.
Responding to his name at crèche now and is playing with other children.
Is making eye contact with other children.

Language is still a problem. He will take his parents hand and grunt and point. But he understands what they say.

Rx. (5) MMR 50M x 2 weekly in water for 3 weeks then report.

18.6.13 No further improvement. Rx. (6) MMR 100M weekly.
30.7.13 Slight improvement, but eating habits still poor. Rx. Silica 6x.
2.8.13 Repeat powder.
12.9.13 Saw a naturopath who said he had a leaky gut. They will try a gluten/dairy free diet. Rx. (7) MMR 500M weekly.

25.10.13 3rd consultation

August - was officially diagnosed with ASD. Having speech and occupational therapy, plus seeing a dietician.

Since they started in March there has been a huge improvement in his communication. Eye contact has improved. He now cuddles his little sister.

He is doing speech therapy 1/7 and childcare 2/7.

Main issues: (a) still no speech, but understands. (b) eating – still wants limited food, mainly carbs. But will eat a lot of what he likes. The big improvement is socialising.

Rx. (8) MMR MM weekly. Nutritional powder.

20.10.14 4th consultation

Was diagnosed ASD on 15.8.13.

Now is a lot more outgoing.
Eye contact better.
Creche 2/7, speech pathology 1/7. Early intervention every 2 weeks.

Is now putting a few words together. Using words appropriately.
Interaction is improving.
Was giving (8) weekly - but less over the last month or so.

Is now counting from 1 to 12., doing jigsaws and saying the alphabet.
Dark around the eyes.

Rx. (9) MMR 10MM every 2 weeks.

+

PART 2: Results

This Part examines the results of my data collection regarding vaccine injured children to 31/12/2022.

It can be read on its own, or in sequence with the remainder of the book if you prefer.

Whilst all data is updated, there are two new vaccine profiles added in this edition – for the Meningococcal meningitis vaccine, and for the MMRV vaccine.

2.6 How Effective was the Treatment of Vaccine Injured Children?

Table 10 shows the classification of results for the 818 cases used in the analysis, and the numeric summary of results for all periods ending **31/12/2022**.

Table 10: Summary of Results from 1989 to December 2022

Summary of Results	Total Results	
	2022	
KEY	#	%
T1 = Strong improvement	171	20.90%
T2 = Improvement	258	31.54%
T3 = No improvement	34	4.16%
T4 = Patient worse	9	1.10%
T5 = Result unclear	162	19.80%
T6 = No follow up	163	19.93%
T7 = Reaction, no follow up	21	2.57%
	818	**100.00%**
Results Excluding No Follow Up		
T1 = Strong improvement	171	26.97%
T2 = Improvement	258	40.69%
T3 = No improvement	34	5.36%
T4 = Patient worse	9	1.42%
T5 = Result unclear	162	25.55%
	634	**100.00%**

Unfortunately, I did not keep all of my early case records from 1986 to the early 1990's, but what is presented will tell a reliable story.

These results have become, for me, a lesson in patient follow-up given that in around 40% of the cases, no analysis was possible since the results were either unclear, or there was no effective follow-up (a decade ago the combined figure was 48.9%, so it is improving).

One reason for a lack of follow-up is that I have many patients who travel for hours to see me, and whilst I ask them to keep in touch by email, and I post out remedies as needed, the fact that I am not readily accessible makes follow-up less straightforward.

Another reason for poor follow-up is because many parents of vaccine injured children have been trying various treatments for years before seeing me. They can be physically and emotionally exhausted, and basically feel that if the new approach doesn't produce immediate results, then they will keep searching for something that does provide a quick result.

As you will see from some of the cases, at times results can be immediate and unambiguous, but mostly it takes time for a chronic condition to resolve, and these parents feel they have no time left.

A final reason for poor follow-up is that in some of the cases there may have been an aggravation of symptoms. I always tell parents that this might happen, and in fact usually is a very positive thing as it means the remedy has touched one **cause** of their child's symptoms. But they forget, and because there is no follow-up, I can't remind them and so they decide to discontinue treatment.

Many cases are classified as unclear because they were taken in the few months before the data collection cut-off point, and a clear pattern of response is yet to be established. In some other cases there are things happening – maybe some remedy reactions which include minor changes in symptoms, but not enough to classify as being a definite improvement.

The latest figures include cases up to 31/12/2022, and it can be seen that the percentage of unusable figures has reduced, and the percentage of improvements has increased.

Table 10.5 shows the summary figures broken into 4 decades excluding no follow-up. The classification codes T1 to T5 used for results are shown in Table 10. Once again, the changing pattern of responses is clear. **Since 2010 the percentage of *Strong Improvements* (T1) and *Improvements* (T2) is greater than 70%.**

Table 10.5: Treatment Results over Four Decades to December 2022

Decades	#	T1	T2	T3	T4	T5	Sum
To 1999	101	10.4%	26.9%	10.4%	4.5%	47.8%	100.0%
2000 to 2009	183	19.7%	43.2%	5.3%	2.3%	29.5%	100.0%
2010 to 2019	333	28.3%	43.0%	5.4%	0.7%	22.6%	100.0%
2020 to 2022	201	37.8%	40.4%	3.2%	0.6%	17.9%	100.0%
Total	**818**	**27.0%**	**40.7%**	**5.4%**	**1.4%**	**25.6%**	**100.0%**

Table 11 compares the percentage of cases for different vaccines which showed either strong (T1) or general (T2) improvement, after excluding cases with no follow-up. And Figure 1 shows this graphically. This data shows some interesting results.

By comparing the improvement rate in the earliest half of the data base to that in the latest half it is clear that my success rate for patients who follow-up is improving over time. And so it should, as a therapist gains more experience and, in my case, instigates an improved follow-up system.

The different improvement percentages between *DPT-only*, *MMR-only* and *DPT + MMR* cases is interesting, and suggests that there may be benefit in detoxing both of these vaccines even if the timing of symptom changes suggests one or the other vaccine were more a problem. The low *DPT-only* figure indicates the preponderance of DPT cases in the first half of my practice, whilst MMR cases became more common in the second half.

Table 11: Percentage of Improvement (T1 + T2) for different vaccines, excluding no follow-up (2022)

Measure	Cases	%
All responses (see Table 10)	818	67.7
First half of total data	409	54.3
Second half of total data	409	74.3
DPT-only remedies used	492	39.1
MMR-only remedies used	168	71.6
DPT & MMR remedies used	86	78.2
Hep B cases	14	63.6
Hib cases	10	37.5
HPV cases	35	54.2
Varicella cases	12	70.0
Meningococcal cases	16	78.6
MMRV cases	13	92.3

The difference in improvement percentages between the other vaccines came as a surprise, especially how strong MMRV was compared to Hib cases.

Table 12 shows the coding I have used for different diseases/conditions. This follows a typical homeopathic schema, beginning with the mind, then from the head to extremities, with others at the end. The Table shows the number of patients per disease category, and associated percentages (taken over the total of all diseases in the different vaccine groups), irrespective of treatment result classification and irrespective of whether multiple vaccine potencies were used.

Figure 1: Percentage of Improvement for different vaccines, excluding no follow-up (2022)

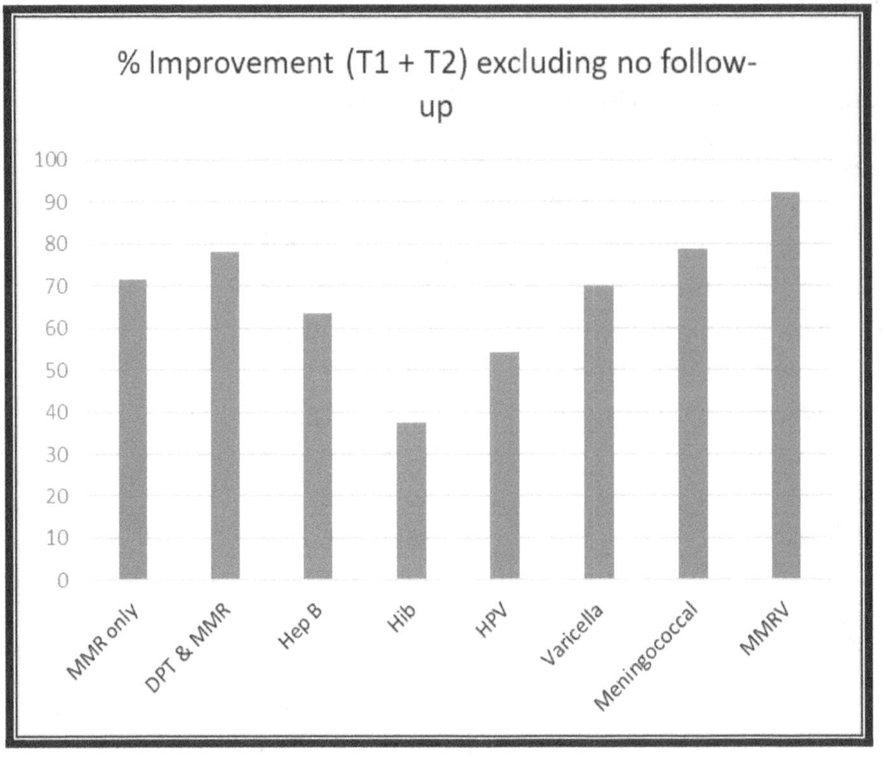

The numbers in Table 12 give the reader an indication of the types of diseases/conditions for which patients presented with the vaccines which appeared to be most involved.

However, there is a lot of detail here which may be studied later as required.

Table 12: Disease Classification and % for Main Vaccines (1)

Code	Symptoms	All DPT	All MMR	Hep B	Hib
	Numbers in each group	**578**	**254**	**14**	**10**
D1	Developmental problems	9.7%	17.7%	7.1%	30.0%
D2	Learning/delayed language	24.9%	62.2%	35.7%	40.0%
D3	Autism/poor interaction	20.6%	63.0%	28.6%	20.0%
D4	AD(H)D type problems	15.1%	14.2%	7.1%	30.0%
D5	Anxiety/stress/bed wetting	14.2%	16.5%	7.1%	0.0%
D6	Epilespy	5.9%	7.1%	7.1%	20.0%
D7	Sleep and associated issues	14.4%	11.0%	7.1%	30.0%
D8	Other neurological problems	9.0%	8.7%	14.3%	20.0%
D9	Other behavioural problems	27.3%	26.0%	21.4%	10.0%
D10	Headaches/Migraines	2.1%	1.6%	0.0%	10.0%
D20	Allergies	13.1%	7.5%	21.4%	0.0%
D26	Sinus/nose poor breathing	5.2%	1.6%	7.1%	20.0%
D28	Throat/neck glands/tonsils/adenoids	8.3%	9.4%	14.3%	10.0%
D30	Asthma	10.6%	3.1%	0.0%	30.0%
D34	Recurring colds/flus/bronch.	13.0%	7.9%	7.1%	20.0%
D38	Other respiratory	3.8%	2.0%	0.0%	10.0%
D40	Ear/hearing problems	13.1%	9.8%	14.3%	10.0%
D50	GIT problems	24.4%	30.7%	42.9%	10.0%
D60	Arthritic/rheumatic	1.7%	2.0%	0.0%	0.0%
D70	Skin problems	37.2%	15.4%	14.3%	40.0%
D80	Screaming/continual crying	4.3%	2.8%	0.0%	0.0%
D84	Weight loss/gain	0.7%	0.8%	0.0%	0.0%
D86	Fevers	2.1%	0.8%	0.0%	0.0%
D88	Listless/energy problems	3.3%	1.6%	7.1%	10.0%
D90	Other problems	4.0%	3.1%	7.1%	0.0%
D92	Acute reactions to vaccines	9.5%	7.1%	14.3%	10.0%

Table 12: Disease Classification and % for Main Vaccines (2)

Code		HPV	Varic.la	Mening	MMRV
	Numbers in each group	**35**	**12**	**16**	**13**
D1	Developmental problems	0.0%	8.3%	12.5%	15.4%
D2	Learning/delayed language	2.9%	75.0%	25.0%	46.2%
D3	Autism/poor interaction	5.7%	91.7%	25.0%	46.2%
D4	AD(H)D type problems	2.9%	16.7%	12.5%	15.4%
D5	Anxiety/stress/bed wetting	25.7%	8.3%	12.5%	15.4%
D6	Epilespy	2.9%	8.3%	6.3%	7.7%
D7	Sleep and associated issues	8.6%	0.0%	12.5%	15.4%
D8	Other neurological problems	22.9%	8.3%	12.5%	15.4%
D9	Other behavioural problems	14.3%	58.3%	25.0%	23.1%
D10	Headaches/Migraines	20.0%	0.0%	0.0%	0.0%
D20	Allergies	5.7%	8.3%	12.5%	0.0%
D26	Sinus/nose poor breathing	0.0%	0.0%	0.0%	0.0%
D28	Throat/neck glands/tonsils/adenoids	0.0%	8.3%	12.5%	15.4%
D30	Asthma	0.0%	8.3%	0.0%	0.0%
D34	Recurring colds/flus/bronch.	2.9%	8.3%	12.5%	15.4%
D38	Other respiratory	0.0%	0.0%	6.3%	7.7%
D40	Ear/hearing problems	2.9%	0.0%	18.8%	0.0%
D50	GIT problems	14.3%	41.7%	37.5%	30.8%
D60	Arthritic/rheumatic	5.7%	0.0%	0.0%	0.0%
D70	Skin problems	11.4%	8.3%	25.0%	30.8%
D80	Screaming/continual crying	0.0%	8.3%	0.0%	0.0%
D84	Weight loss/gain	0.0%	8.3%	0.0%	0.0%
D86	Fevers	0.0%	0.0%	0.0%	0.0%
D88	Listless/energy problems	5.7%	0.0%	0.0%	0.0%
D90	Other problems	31.4%	0.0%	6.3%	0.0%
D92	Acute reactions to vaccines	14.3%	16.7%	6.3%	0.0%

2.7 Symptom Profiles of Eight Vaccines

The symptom profiles for the eight main vaccines studied will now be presented, together with other analyses based on the data.

It should be noted that these profiles are attempts to find a common group of symptoms likely to be produced by each vaccine. **It does not mean that every symptom will appear in every patient, or that patients will only produce symptoms in the profile.** Further, whilst the numbers are slowing growing for the Hep B, HPV, Varicella, Hib, Meningococcal and MMRV profiles, extra data is needed to establish more exact findings.

However, if reliable profiles can be developed, this will assist practitioners and parents to recognise potential blocks to successful treatment.

2.7(a) Symptom Profile of the DPT Vaccine

In order to further analyse the change in the nature of the DPT based vaccines as they have expanded from the original 3-valent vaccine (DPT or DTPw) to a six-valent vaccine *Infanrix HEXA* (which is sometimes called DPT HEXA), I divided the data into three groups. These are different to the three time periods discussed earlier, which just happened to be when data was updated and occurred both during and at the end of the years mentioned.

The three new time periods and the corresponding changes in the DPT vaccines are shown in Table 13. It was assumed that the relevant time-period began 3 years after the introduction of the new vaccine.

This is not exact as some patients would have the old vaccine due to presenting earlier than average, or because their doctors were using up old stocks. The different time-based groups cover:

Period 1: DTPw - [Diphtheria + Tetanus + Pertussis (whole cell)].
Period 2: DTPa+ - [D + T + Pertussis (acellular) + Hib and/or Hep B and/or IPV (polio)].
Period 3: Infanrix HEXA - [D + T + P(a) + Hib + HepB + IPV] or DPT HEXA

Remember that the data classification is: T1 = Strong improvement; T2 = Improvement; T3 = No improvement; T4 = Patient worse; T5 = Result unclear; T6 = No follow up; T7 = Reaction, then no follow up

It is immediately clear how much more successful treatment was in each succeeding period (T1 + T2 = 32.3%; 53.8%; 69.3% - after the removal of no follow-up cases T6). This is almost certainly more a result of improved treatment resulting from greater experience and follow-up than the expanding vaccines being easier to treat.

This data will be examined again in Figure 3 following.

Table 13: Results in Three Periods Showing DTP Changes to 2022 (excluding no follow up) – Numbers of patients and percentages

Years	Vaccine	T1	T2	T3	T4	T5	T7	Sum
1987 - 1999	DTPw	6	15	7	3	31	3	65
	%	9.2%	23.1%	10.8%	4.6%	47.7%	4.6%	**100%**
2000 - 2008	DTPa + misc	18	32	6	3	29	5	**93**
	%	19.4%	34.4%	6.5%	3.2%	31.2%	5.4%	100.0%
2009 - 2022	DTPa Hexa	63	93	12	1	50	6	**225**
	%	28.0%	41.3%	5.3%	0.4%	22.2%	2.7%	**100%**
Total	#	87	140	25	7	110	14	**383**
	%	22.7%	36.6%	6.5%	1.8%	28.7%	3.7%	**100%**

The analysis presented in Figure 2 (below) indicates that the four main groups of symptoms related to injury by the DPT group vaccines are mental/emotional disorders, gastrointestinal (GIT) problems, a range of respiratory diseases, and skin conditions. Behavioural and learning problems are significant, especially learning and anger issues. Asthma and recurring respiratory infections and GIT problems are also major issues. Eczema staring around 2, 4 or 6 months is common.

NOTE: *In the clinic, many practitioners have noticed a common progression of a healthy infant who develops eczema or a related skin condition following vaccination. The skin is "cured" with cortisone creams, and then after some time the child develops asthma. If the asthma is treated successfully then in such cases the skin eruption will always return for a period of time, before the patient is completely cured. In fact, if the skin condition does not return in such a case, the practitioner knows that the job is unfinished.*

We can see that the DPT based vaccines are a very likely cause of such a history, and potencies of the vaccine should be considered as part of the treatment program.

A new analysis is presented in Figure 2.5 which looks at how the overall DPT figures change when looked at in three different ways:
(1) symptom profiles of all patients who were given the remedies to detox the different DPT vaccines since 1985;
(2) symptom profiles of patients who initially were given **only** the DPT remedies (very little difference apart from more developmental issues); and
(3) the symptoms pictures of patients who were initially prescribed **both** DPT and MMR detox remedies (not taken at the same time) where the differences are significantly more psychological issues, and fewer skin and respiratory issues.

Figure 2: Symptom Profile of the DPT Vaccine

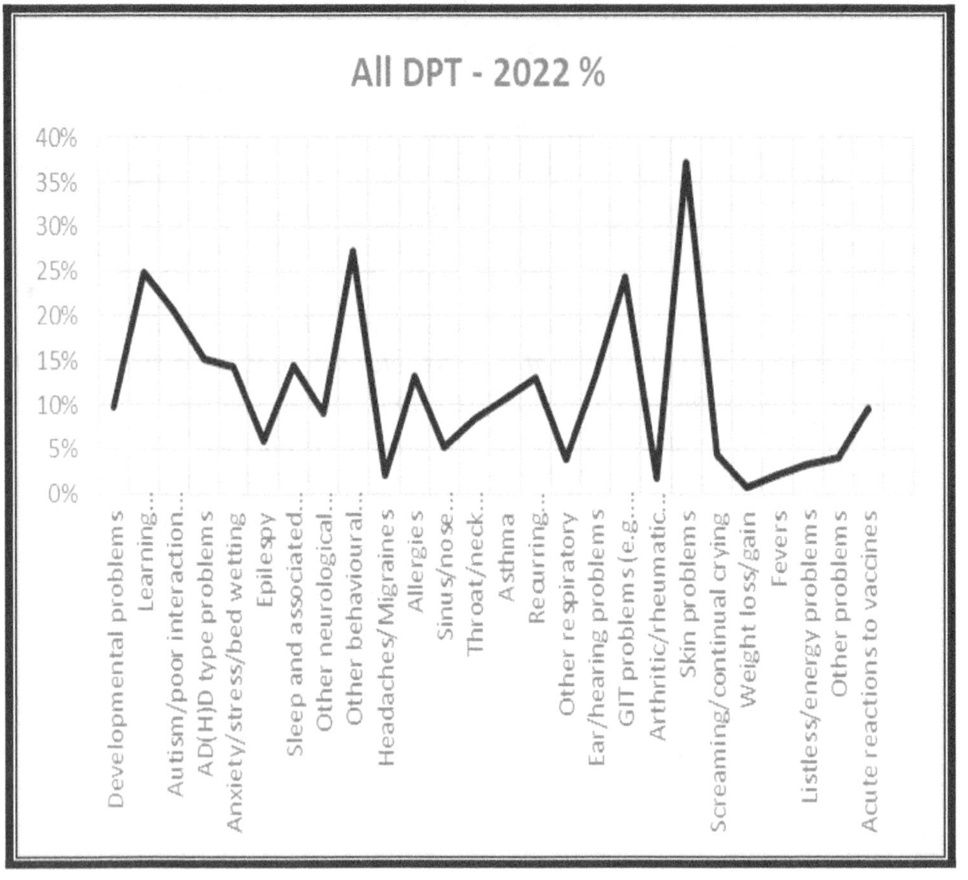

The findings arising from the data presented in Figure 2.5 are not unexpected as it will be shown below that the MMR picture is very different from the DPT picture especially in the psychological, skin and respiratory areas.

Figure 2.5: Different Data Collections for DPT Files

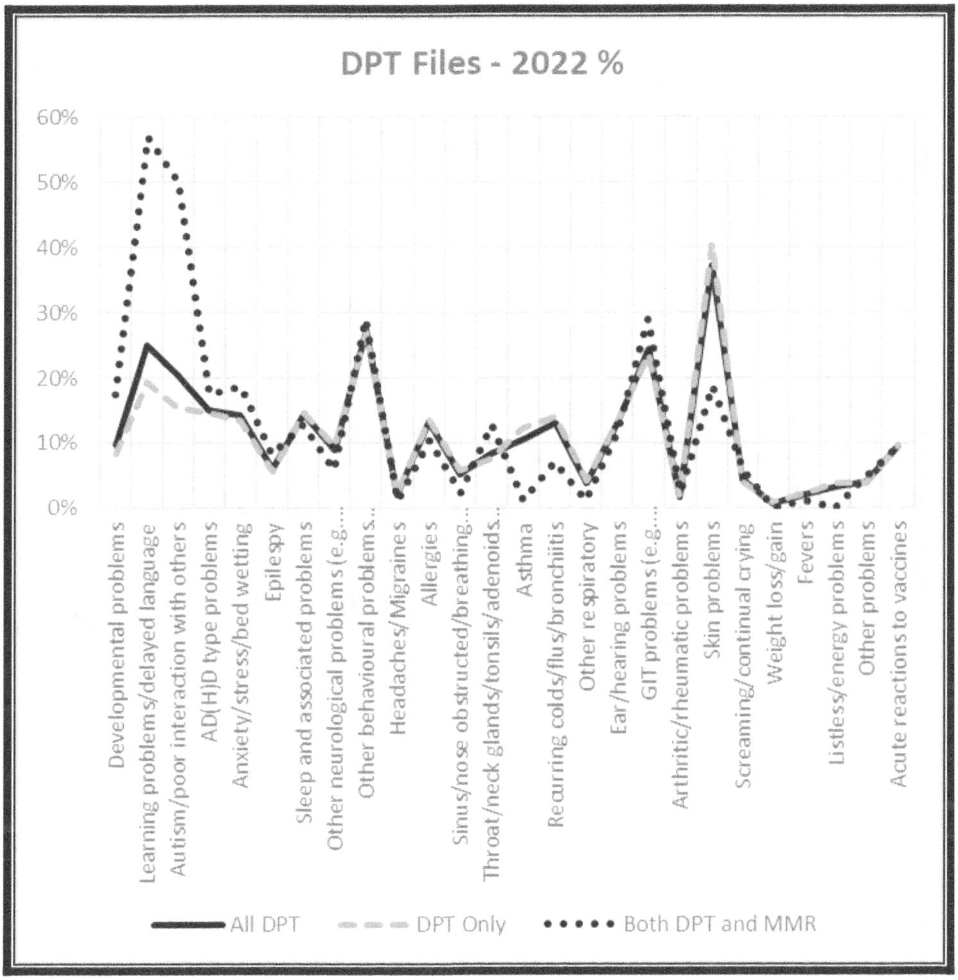

The data presented in Figure 3 shows the DPT figures split across the 3 time periods which roughly correspond to the use of the 3 different types of DPT vaccines (DTPw; DTPa +; Infanrix Hexa).

Figure 3: Symptom Profile of DPT for 3 Different Vaccines

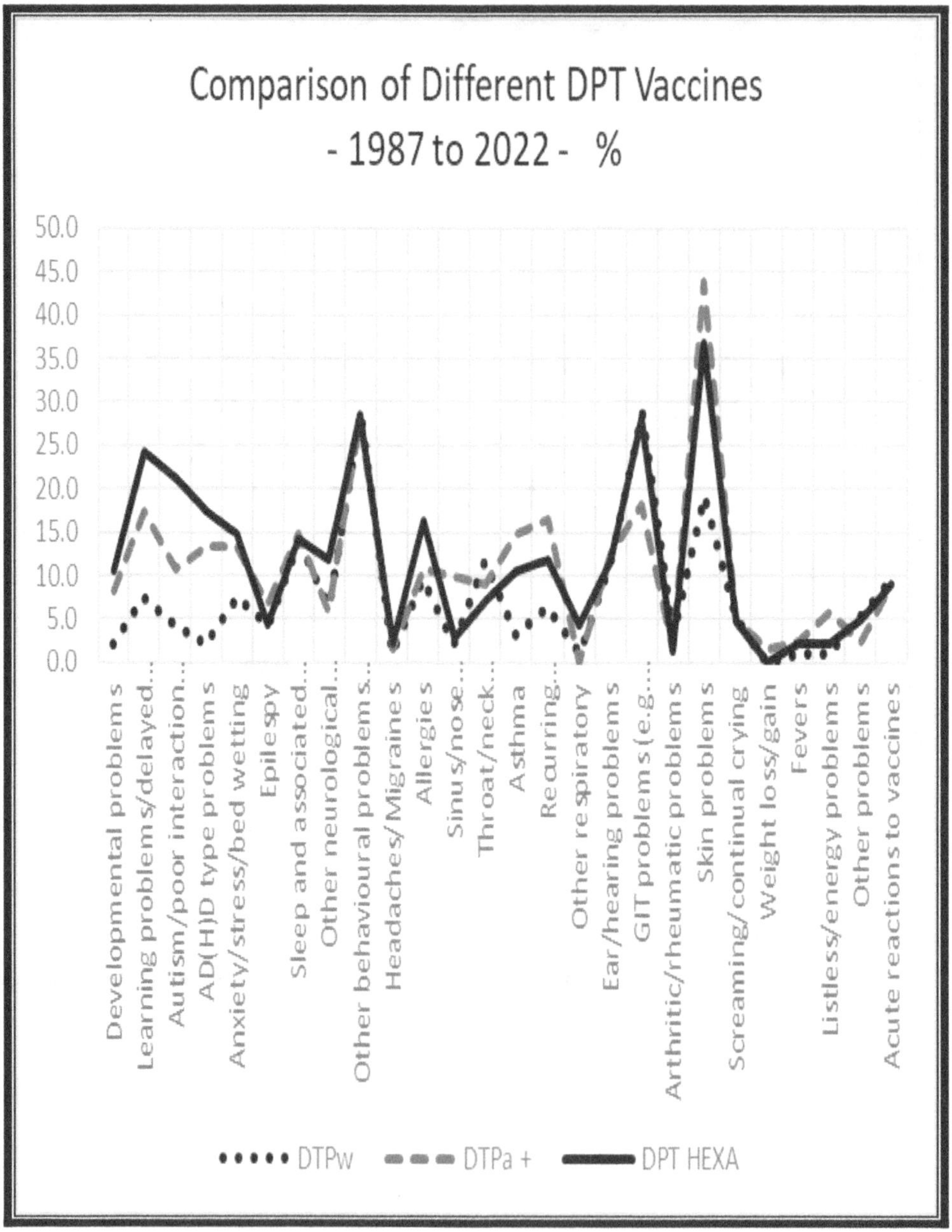

NOTE: Percentage figures, unless otherwise stated, show the % of patients in each cohort with the defined condition – e.g. around 37% of all DPT HEXA patients have/had a skin condition.

It is apparent from Figure 3 that whilst the physical profile of the changing DPT vaccines has remained broadly similar (there are now more allergies and GIT issues), there has been a clear increase in developmental, learning, behavioural as well as neurological issues. The pertussis component was changed from whole cell (Pw) to acellular (Pa) to reduce potential complications from the vaccine, even though Pa was not as effective as Pw.

However this data suggests that as the number of antigens has increased from 3 in the old DPT vaccine to 4, 5 and now 6 in the current HEXA vaccine, that there has been a steady increase in developmental, learning, behavioural as well as neurological issues. This analysis is continued in Section 2.8 (c) and 2.8(d).

Some parents attempt to split the HEXA vaccine into fewer antigens per needle, but the problem with this is that the child then receives two or three times the amount of aluminium, formaldehyde, etc etc which can no doubt cause additional complications.

2.7(b) Symptom Profile of the MMR Vaccine

Figure 4 shows the symptom profile (%) of the MMR vaccine at both 2014 and 2022. There is little change apart from somewhat less autism and somewhat more other behavioural problems. As well, the MMR vaccine seems to be associated with a significant number of GIT problems at both time periods.

Given the controversy sparked by Dr Wakefield's well publicised findings suggesting a link between MMR vaccine, gut disorders and

autism, these findings may not surprise many readers. They do in fact reinforce Dr Wakefield's conclusions from a totally different analytical perspective.
In my own clinic I have tended to assume that the more "in your face" ADHD type of behaviour was related to the DPT vaccine, and the more withdrawn or autistic type of behaviour more related to the MMR vaccine. The analysis in fact shows that the MMR vaccine can be related to both, and in the previous Section it showed that DPT HEXA can also be associated with learning/developmental/ ASD type behaviour.

So, the combination of behavioural/learning/delayed language/GIT problems indicates that a potency of the MMR vaccine may be of great value in treatment.

Figure 4: Symptom Profile of the MMR Vaccine

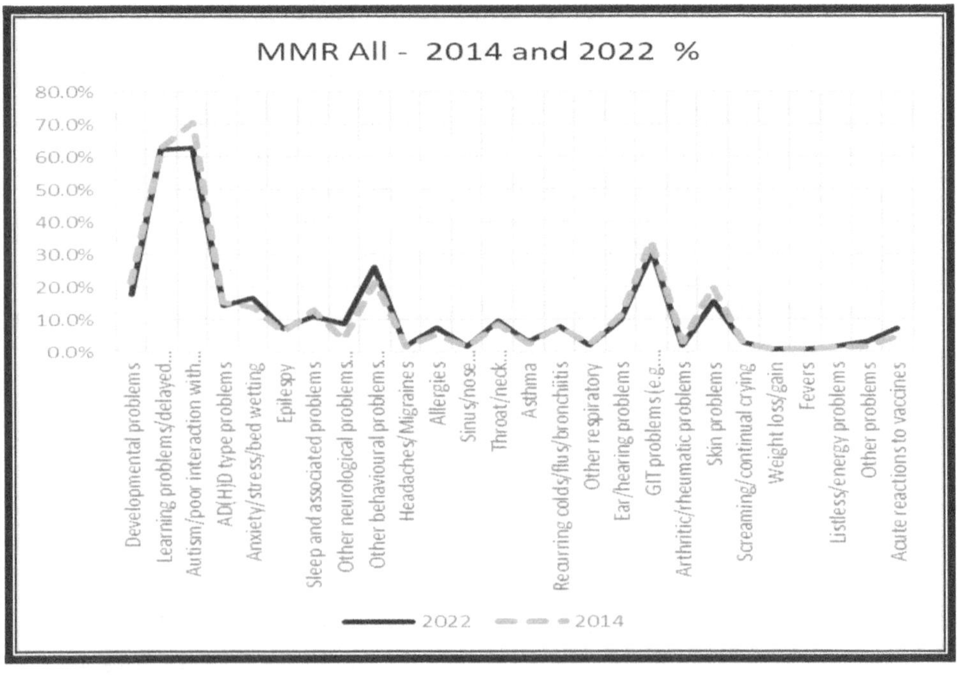

Note that when a comparison was made between the percentages for *all MMR* cases and *MMR-only* cases, the figures were nearly identical (unlike with DPT).

Also remember that because of the universal nature of the *Law/Principle of Similars*, the remedy can be used in UNvaccinated children who present with that symptom complex (this applies the other vaccine potencies as well).

The difference between the MMR and DPT HEXA vaccines is highlighted in Figure 5 which compares the MMR and the DPT HEXA percentages of symptoms to the total group.

Figure 5: Comparison of MMR and DPT HEXA Group Percentages

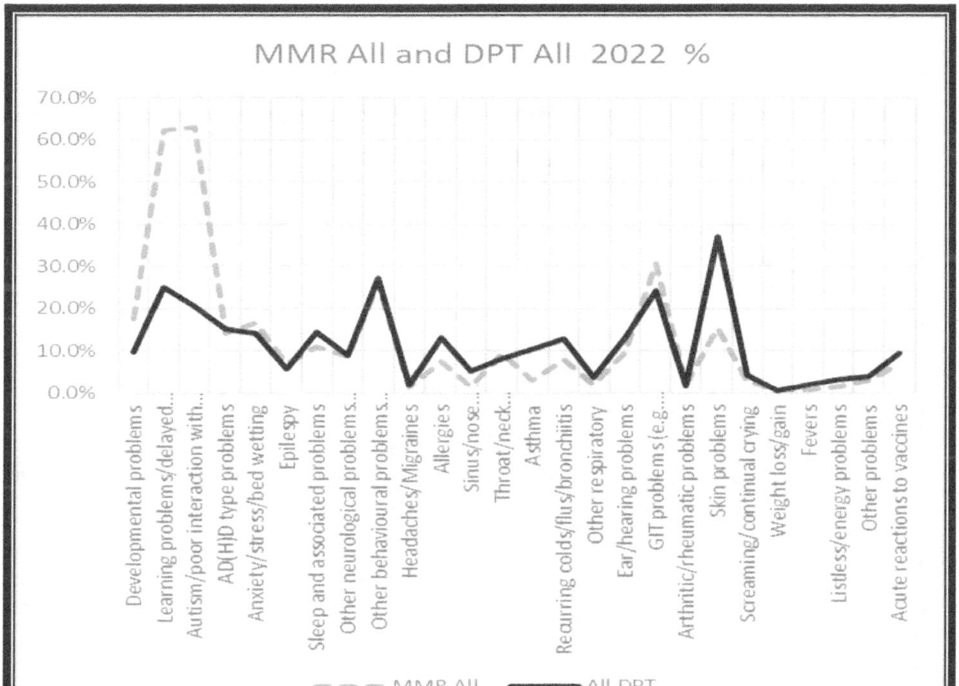

Despite the higher percentage of learning/language/social interaction symptoms in the DPT HEXA group than in previous DPT vaccines, it is still significantly below the MMR figures. DPT HEXA still has a greater percentage of skin issues than MMR, but interestingly it now has a similar percentage of GIT issues (previously the MMR percentage was much higher than DPT).

2.7(c) Symptom Profile of the Hepatitis B Vaccine

The symptom profiles for the Hepatitis B vaccine in Figure 6 and the Hib vaccine in Figure 7 are based on small sample sizes (14 and 10 patients respectively), and the conclusions drawn are therefore less certain than for the DPT and MMR vaccines.

Figure 6: Symptom Profile of the Hep B vaccine

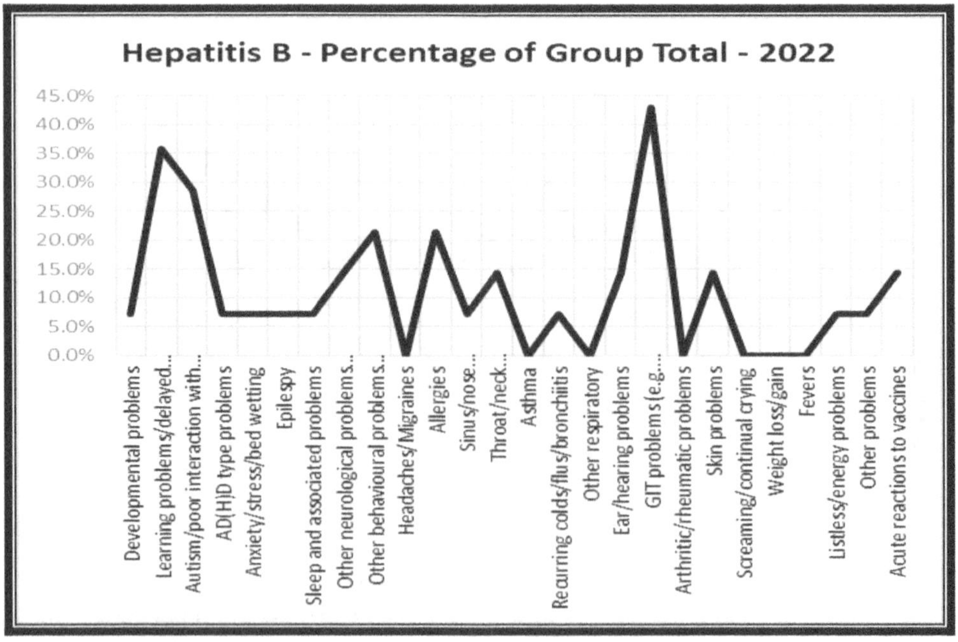

The impact of GIT problems in the Hepatitis B profile may be expected since the disease itself is an inflammation of the liver, with subsequent GIT consequences. It is possible that the vaccine causes injury in the area it is attempting to protect (a not uncommon consequence of pharmaceutical medicine in many areas).

2.7(d) Symptom Profile of the Hib Vaccine

The Haemophilus Influenza type B (Hib) vaccine profile shown in Figure 7 is an interesting one, providing as it does another combination of respiratory and skin problems with some learning, language and ADHD type issues. Compared to the DPT vaccine, we find relatively more respiratory problems, and similar skin problems (see Figure 13.5 below). This once again may be an example of a vaccine causing problems in an area which it is meant to protect, given that Hib is a respiratory related condition.

Figure 7: Symptom Profile of the Hib Vaccine

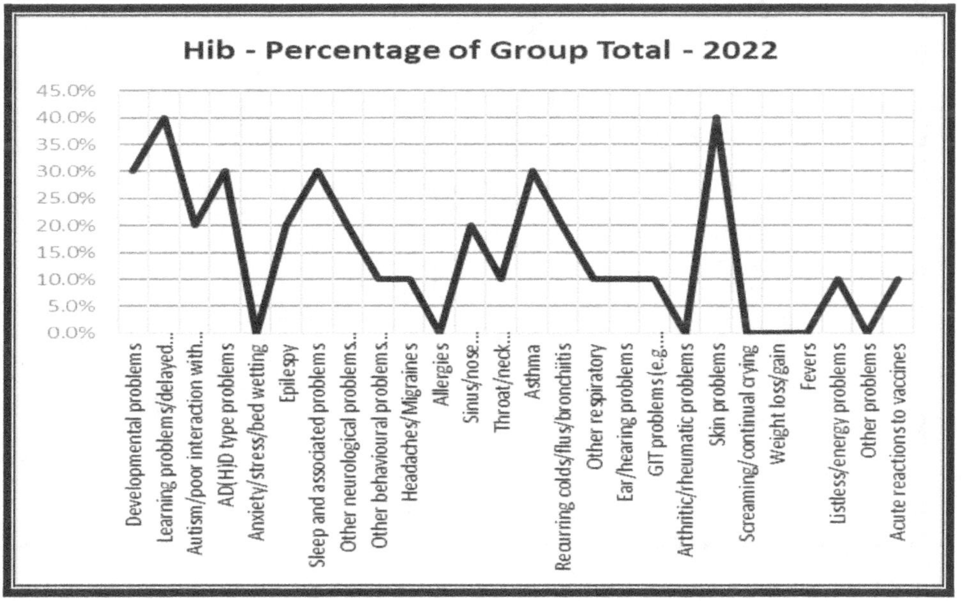

2.7(e) Symptom Profile of the Varicella Vaccine

The symptom profile of the Varicella vaccine is shown in Figure 8. It is based on only 12 patients, but the symptom percentages of the Varicella group are quite remarkable. There is a similarity with the MMR profile in that there are very high percentages of learning, socialisation and general behavioural issues, as well as GIT issues.

It is now possible to identify the impact of the MMRV vaccine, which is now in common use, as the Varicella component could well amplify the MMR-related symptoms. Figure 12 shows this comparison.

Figure 8: Symptom Profile of the Varicella Vaccine

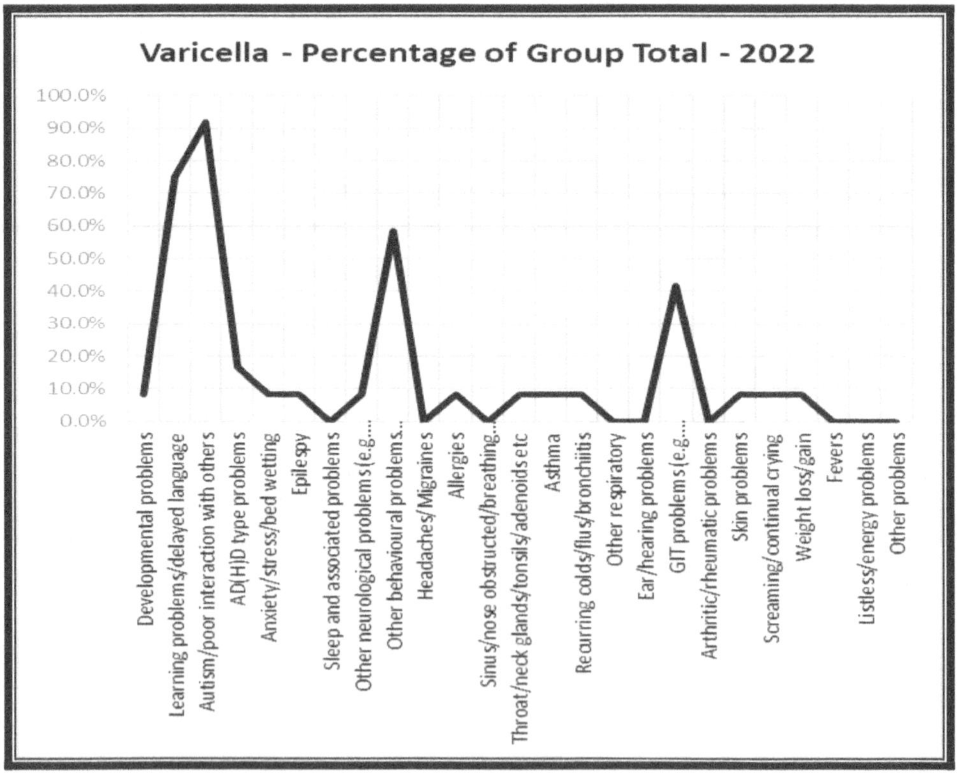

2.7(f) Symptom Profile of the HPV Vaccine

Once again, this is the first analysis I have made of the HPV vaccine, and presented in this new edition. It is drawn from only 11 patients, but shows in Figure 9 a very clear anxiety/neuological picture, plus GIT symptoms. I have seen a lot of neurological impacts from Gardasil so this profile was totally expected.

Figure 9: Symptom Profile of the HPV (Gardasil) Vaccine

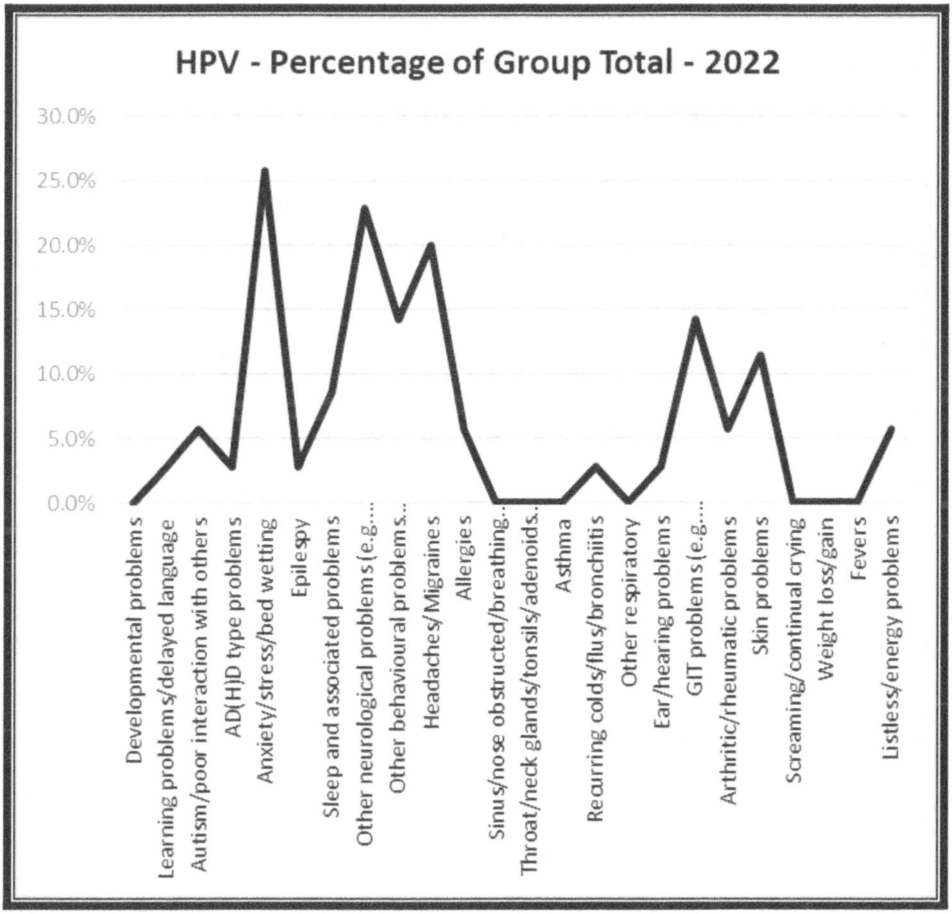

2.7(6) Symptom Profile of the Meningococcal Vaccine

Finally, another new profile for this edition, but drawing from only 6 patients is the Meningococcal profile shown in Figure 10. GIT symptoms dominate the physical symptom profile, and behavioural, learning, and social interaction symptoms are strong, but more data is needed.

Figure 10: Symptom Profile of the Meningococcal Vaccine

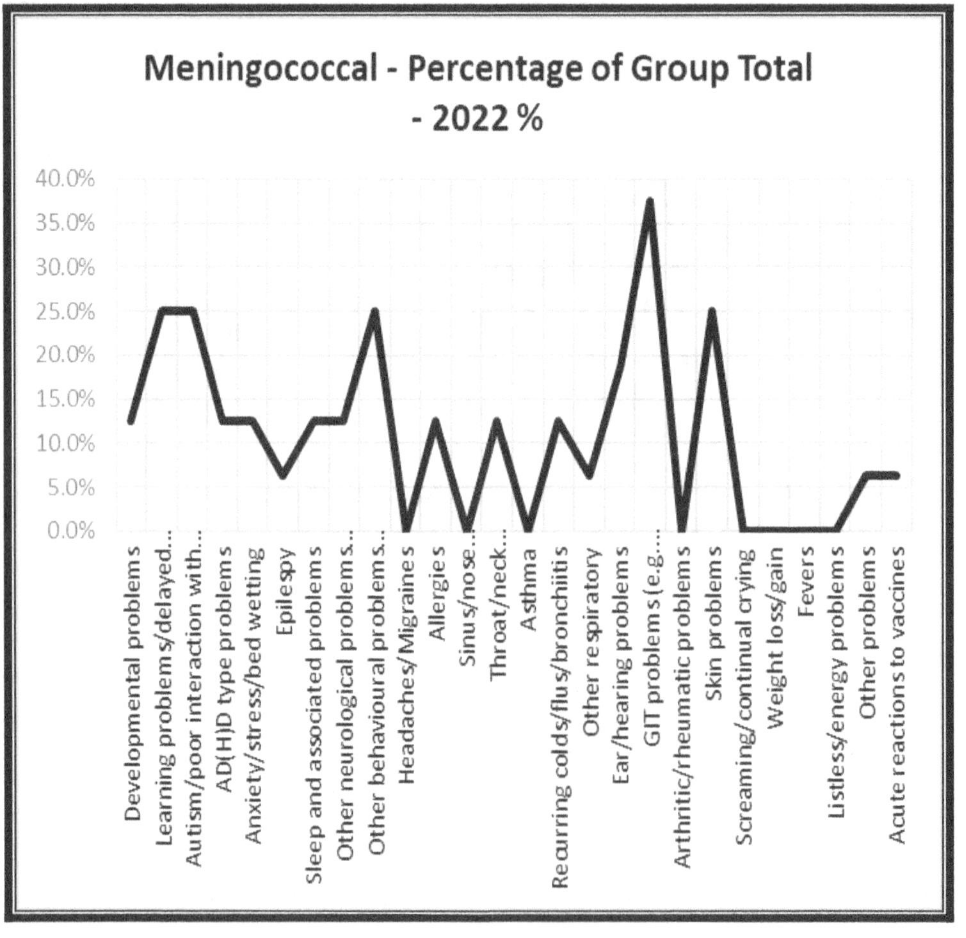

2.7(7) Symptom Profile of the MMRV Vaccine

The use of the MMRV vaccine is now becoming more common. Figure 10.1 below was based on only 12 patients, and the profile may well change as more data is collected.

Figure 12 below contains a comparison of the MMR, Varicella and the MMRV vaccines. This shows a general similarity between most symptoms, apart from general behavioural issues, learning and developmental and ASD issues.

Figure 10.1: Symptom Profile of the MMRV Vaccine

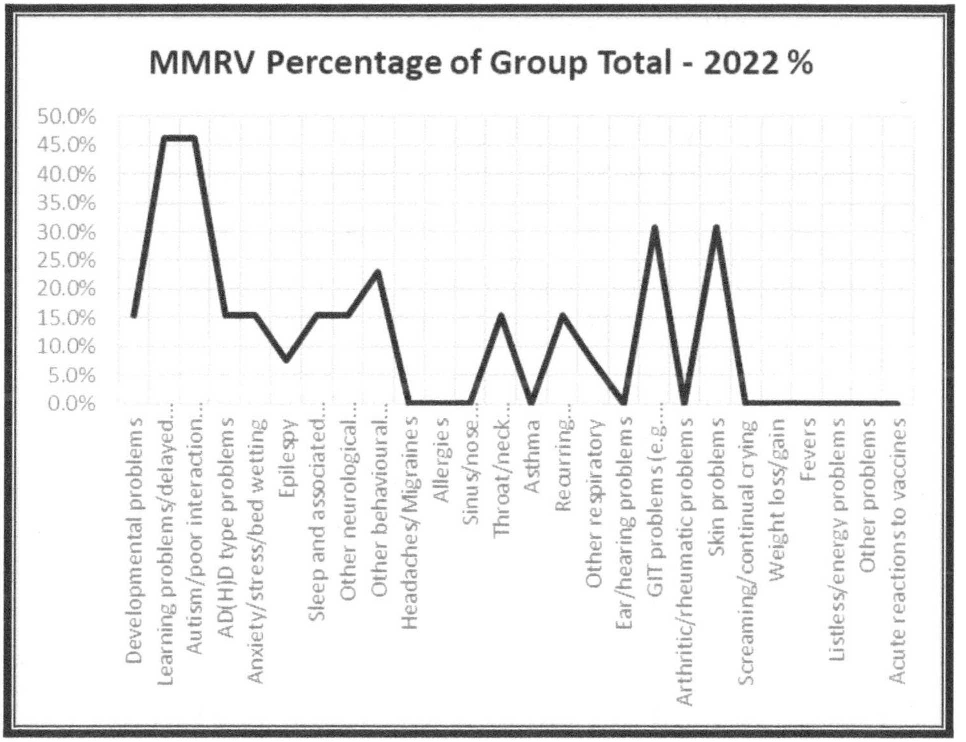

2.7(8) Comparison of Results: All Data V's T1 and T2 Data

The purpose of this new section is to provide a check of how accurate my vaccine symptom profiles have been in previous editions as well as in this edition.

Accuracy will be assessed by examining the symptom profile of all data for a particular vaccine and comparing that to the symptom profile of only cases that have had a positive result – the T1 T2 cases. **IF the two profiles for each vaccine are very similar it means that the symptoms collected whilst taking the case can reliably approximate the symptoms removed by using potencies of the vaccine**, and the previous and current symptoms profiles are reliable.

I am able to now do this in a meaningful way (apart for the Hib vaccine which only recorded a single positive result out of 10 cases) becase the data base has grown over the years and permits this analysis.

I had prepared Tables of data, but I think many readers would have just rolled their eyes and moved on, so instead I have prepared seven small Figures which readily show the differences.

As will be seen from the following seven Figures, the positive results for the DPT, MMR, Varicella and MMRV vaccines are very similar. There are a few significant differences with the HPV, Hepatitis B and Meningococcal vaccines. It is likely (but not certain) that these differences will become fewer as the data collections continue to grow.

Overall, it is reasonable to conclude that the symptom profiles developed for the different vaccines over the years have been reliable and meaningful.

The seven Figures will now follow for those readers interested in this analysis. Remember, **accuracy is guaged by how close the solid lines and the dotted lines are.**

Figure 10.2: Accuracy of DPT Symptom Profiles

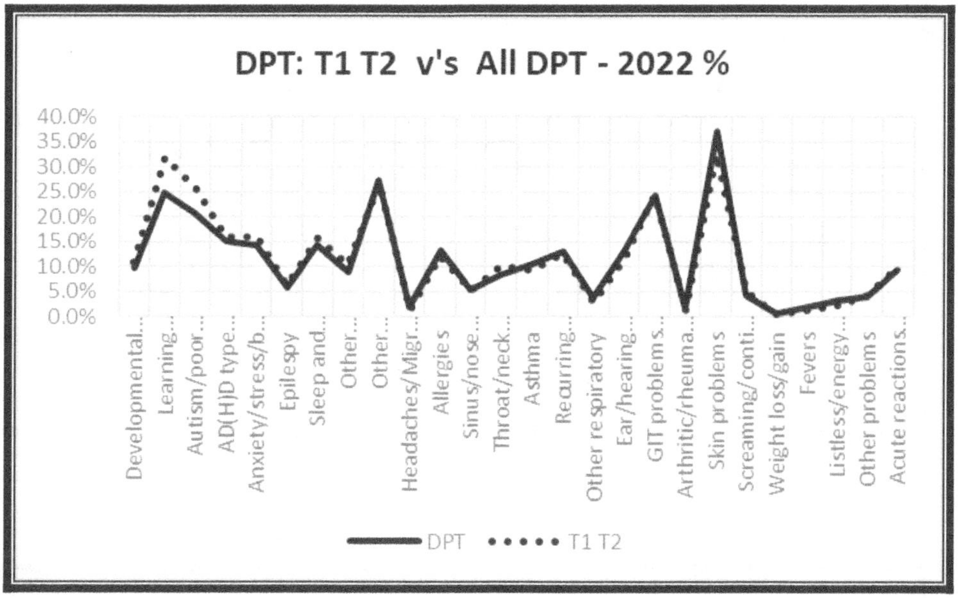

Figure 10.3: Accuracy of MMR Symptom Profiles

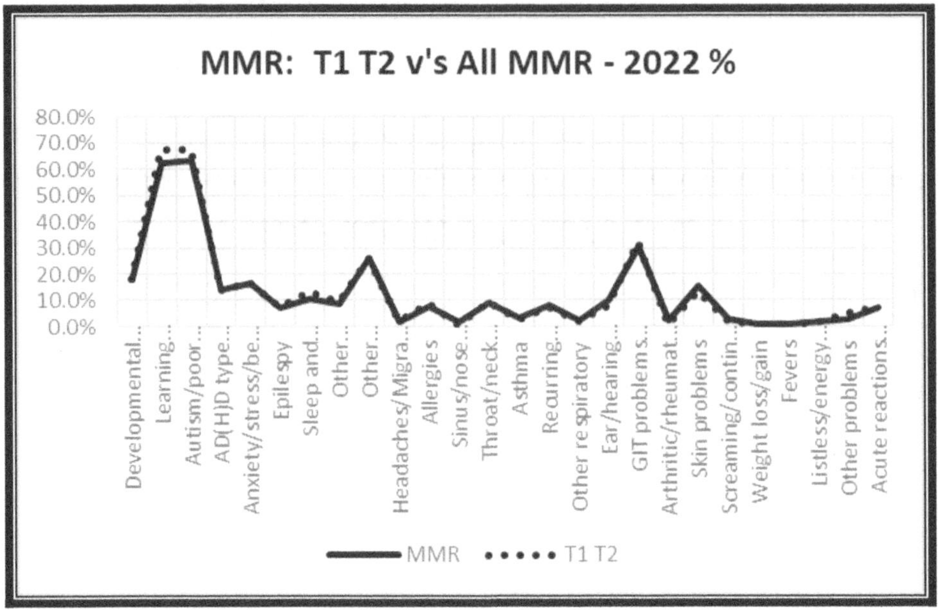

Figure 10.4: Accuracy of Varicella Symptom Profiles

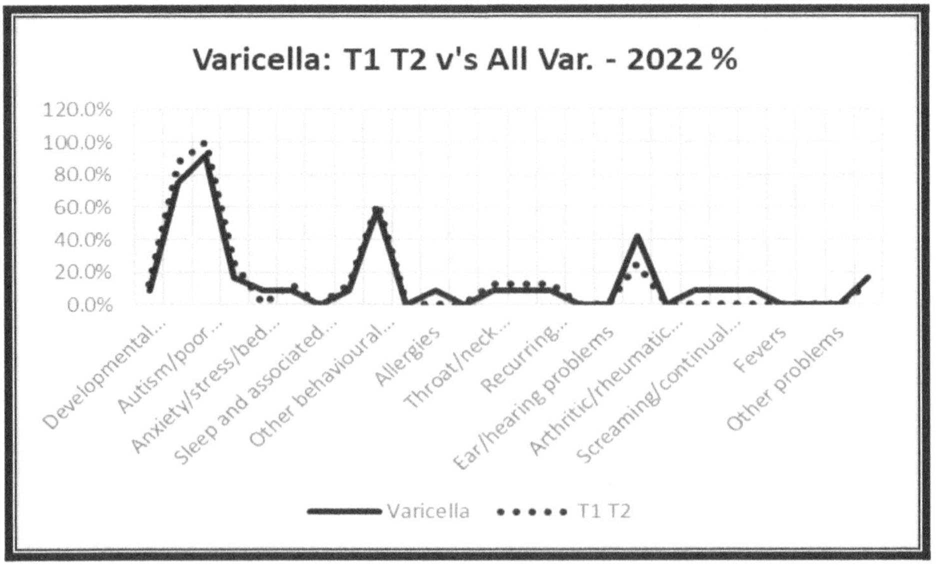

Figure 10.5: Accuracy of MMRV Symptom Profiles

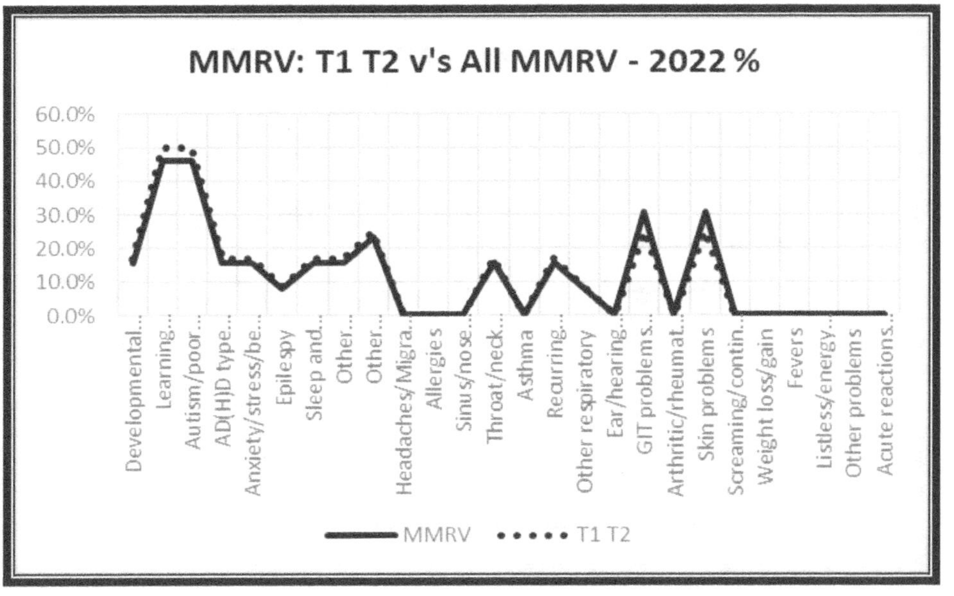

Figure 10.6: Accuracy of HPV Symptom Profiles

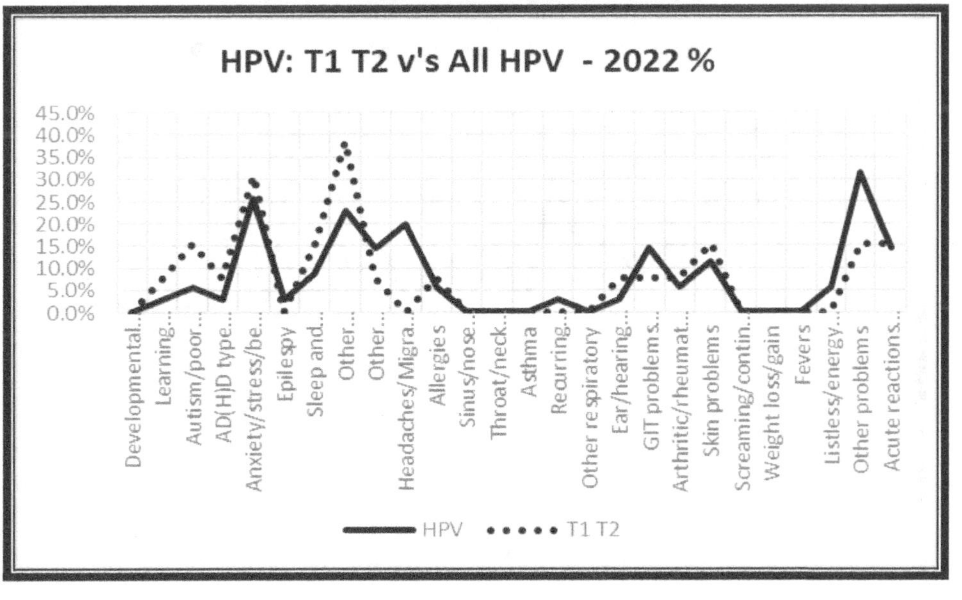

Figure 10.7: Accuracy of Hepatitis B Symptom Profiles

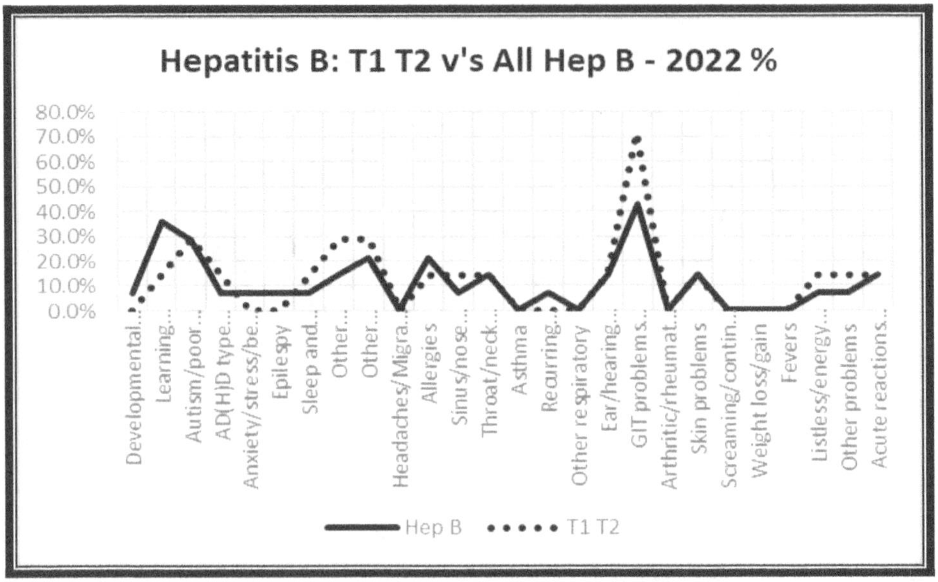

Figure 10.8: Accuracy of Meningococcal Symptom Profiles

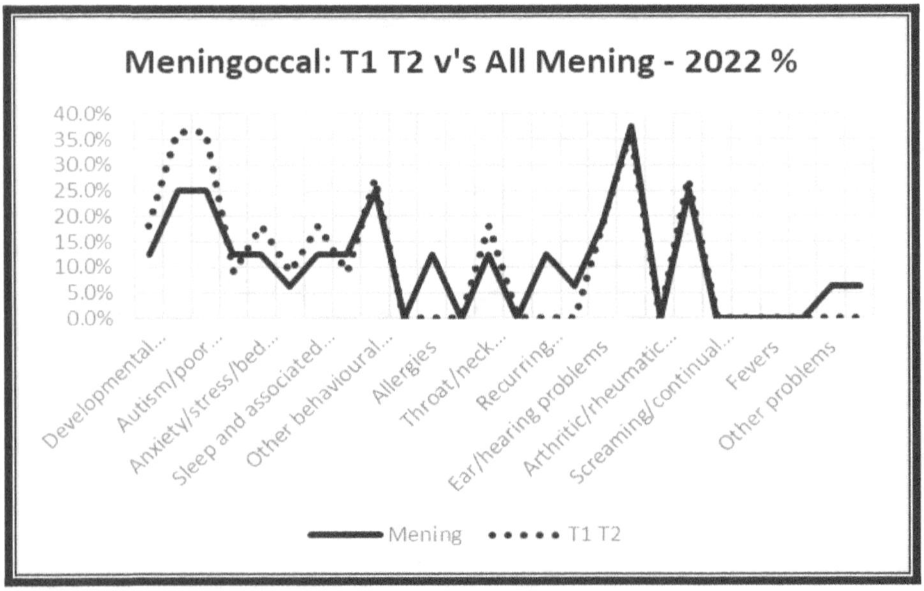

2.8 Comparative Profiles of Vaccines

In practice, much of what any homoeopath will do comes down to comparative analyses – between different possible causes of the patient's problem, and between different remedies that have some "similar" relevance to the case on the level of cause or of symptoms.

The purpose of the next Figures is to assist practitioners, and parents, to differentiate between vaccines to help clarify which vaccine is most likely to be the cause of the injury.

This section is still work in progress. The number of patients involved in the data collection for all but the MMR and DPT groups of vaccines is still relatively small, so the profiles may well change somewhat as the data base increases.

2.8(a) Symptom Comparison of Meningococcal and Gardasil Vaccines + Infanrix HEXA

A comparison of the symptom profiles of the Meningococcal and HPV (Gardasil) vaccines is shown in Figure 11. They were shown together because they had no obvious connection with the DPT group or MMR group of vaccines.

The two symptom profiles show few similarities. However, when the Infanrix HEXA vaccine is included, there is quite a consistency with Meningococcal vaccine. This may suggest that when the two vaccines are given at the same time the child will get a "double whammy" of effect.

Figure 11: Comparison of Meningococcal, Gardasil and HEXA Vaccines

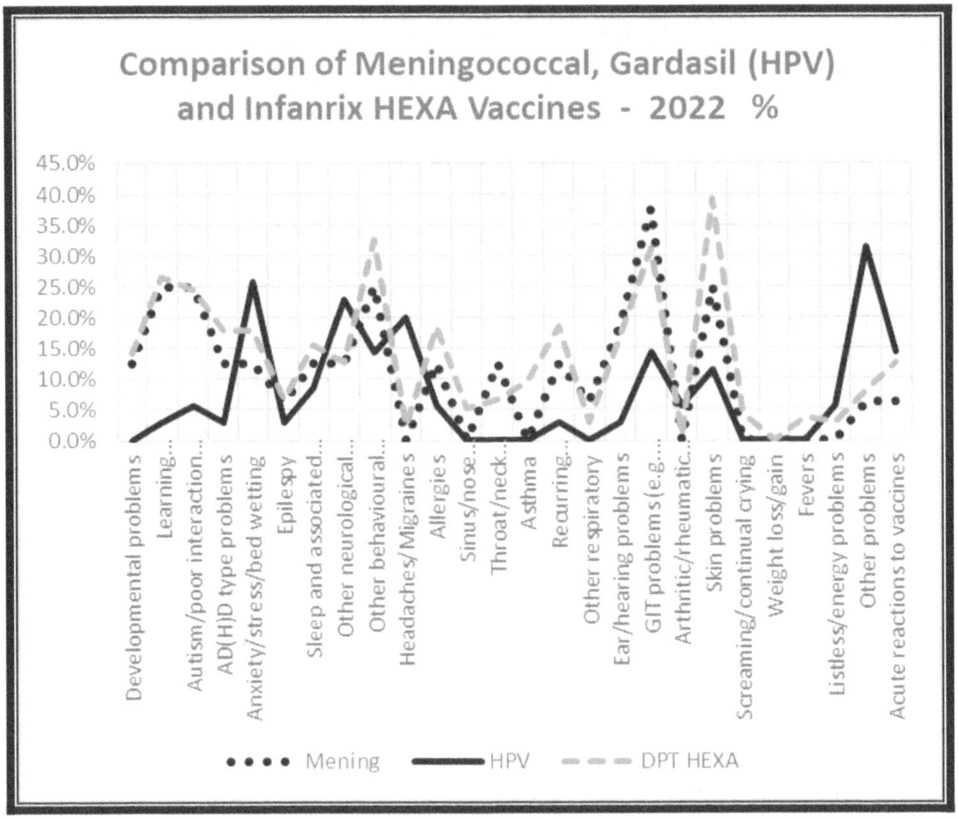

2.8(b) Symptom Comparison of MMR, MMRV and Varicella Vaccines

Figure 12 shows similarities between the symptom profiles of the MMR vaccine and the Varicella (Chicken Pox) vaccine. In this edition it has been possible to provide a profile of the MMRV vaccine for the first time (see also Figure 10.5 above), and this shows similarities with the other two vaccines. The learning/speech/autism symptoms appear to be less than expected (but based on a small patient sample), and skin symptoms more than expected. As the data base grows over time it will be interesting to see how the symptom relationships change, if at all, and one would have expected the MMRV profile to have been between MMR and V profiles.

Figure 12: Symptom Comparison of MMR, MMRV and Varicella Vaccines

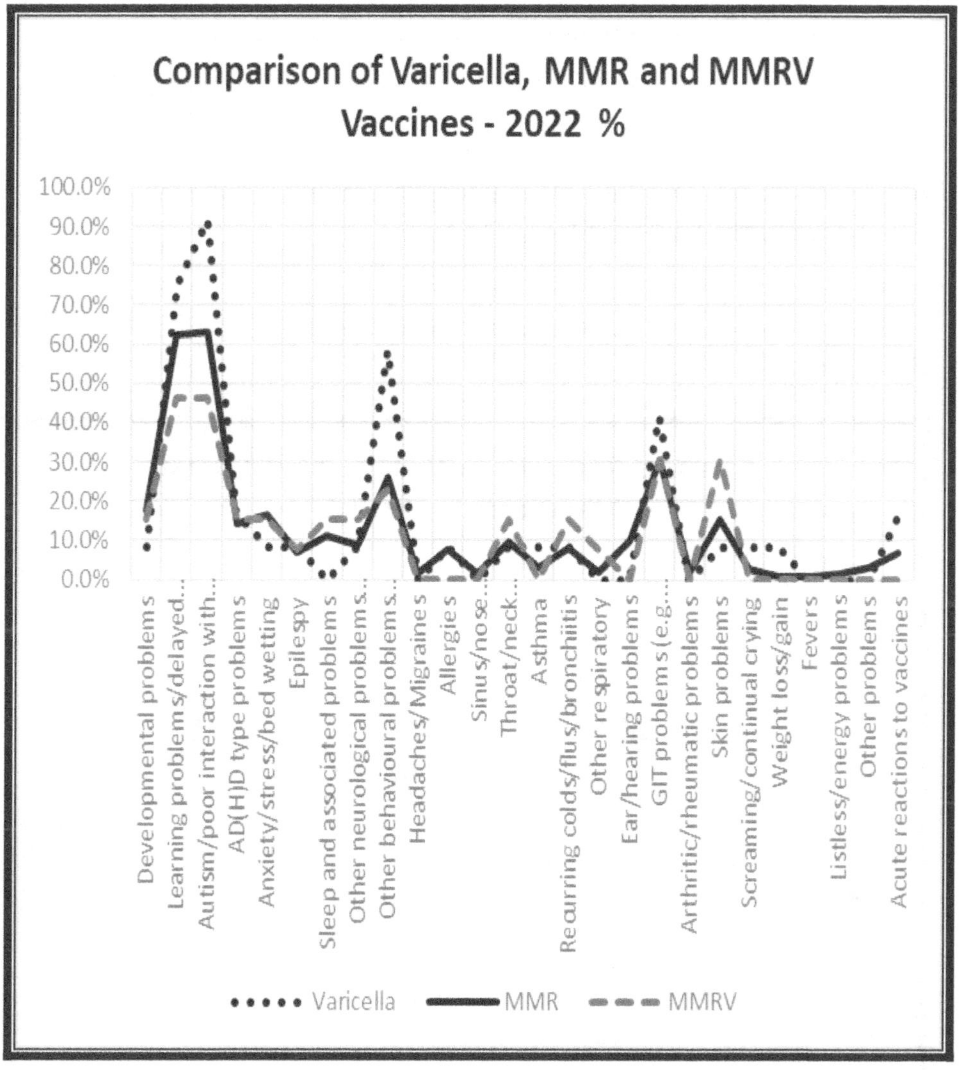

2.8(c) Symptom Comparison of the original DTPw vaccine and the Hepatitis B and Haemophilus type b (Hib) vaccines

Figure 3 above shows the difference between the original DTPw vaccine and the current Infanrix HEXA vaccine. Figure 13 compares the DTPw vaccine (before more antigens were added), Hepatitis B and Haemophilus Influenzae type b (Hib) vaccines. This comparison has relevance because Hep B and Hib are components of the current Infanrix HEXA vaccine (which also includes DTPa and Polio antigens).

Emotionally and intellectually similarities are seen in the "other behavioural" area, but not elsewhere. Physically, there are GIT similarities with Hep B but few with Hib.

Figure 13: Symptoms Comparison of the original DTPw, Hep B and Hib Vaccines

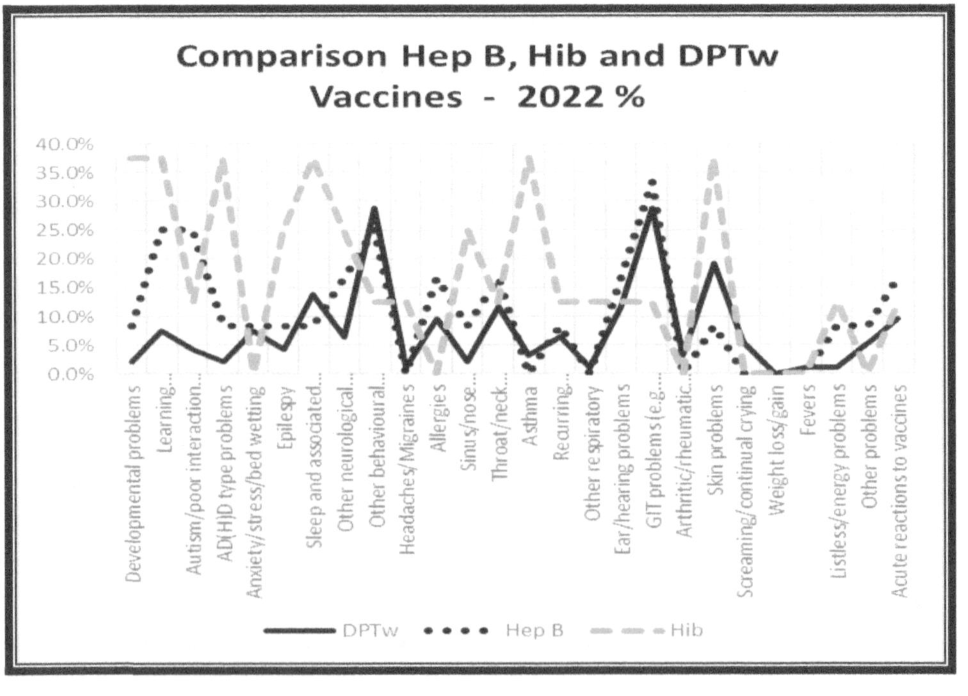

This gives some insight into the pressures that led to the symptom changes between DTPw and Infanrix Hexa.

2.8(d) Symptoms Comparison of Infanrix HEXA, Hep B, Hib and DTPw vaccines

Figure 13.5 introduces Infanrix Hexa with DTPw and the Hib and Hep B vaccines, we see that the old DTPw profile has changed to cover a greater percentage of emotional and intellectual symptoms.

It would appear reasonable to suggest that one effect of adding the Hib and Hep B antigens to create the new Infanrix HEXA vaccine (effectively DTPa + Polio + Hib + Hep B), is to change the emotional and intellectual profile considerably as can be seen in Figure 13.5.

Unfortunately, a symptom profile for the Polio component is not available as it would be interesting to see what effect it may have had.

The physical profile has changed from DTPw to Infanrix HEXA, but less so. Gastrointentinal (GIT) issues affect the same percentage of respondents, and some other percentages are similar, but in general HEXA has caused more people to have more health issues that the old "triple antigen" DTPw.

Figure 13.5: Symptoms Comparison of Infanrix HEXA, Hepatitis B, Hib and DTPw Vaccines

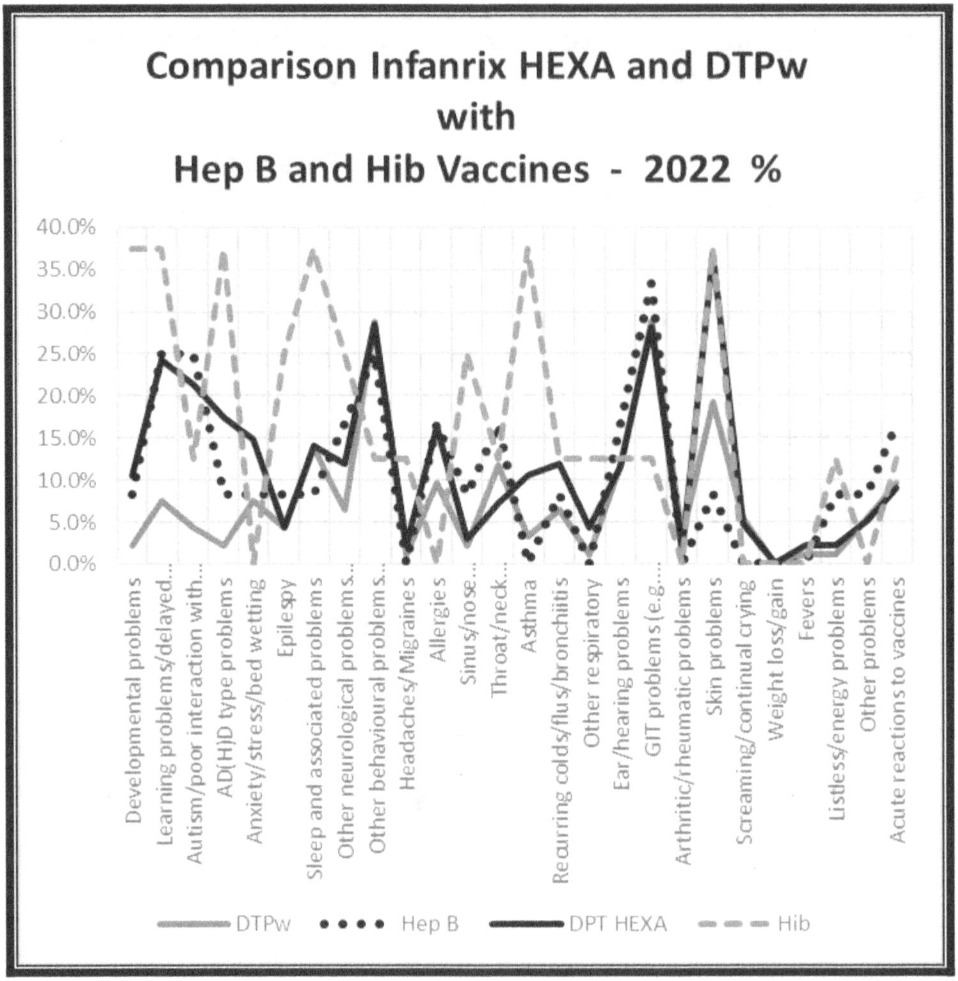

2.9 Comparative Analysis of Disease Groupings

Another way to compare the differences in symptom groupings between the different vaccines is to further group symptoms under the following six general headings: developmental and behavioural problems; neurological problems; respiratory/ENT; GIT; skin; other.

This data differs from earlier Graphs and Tables in that **it looks at the total number of symptoms recorded and strikes percentages to this total number**. This is why, for example, the percentage of GIT symptoms which is around 30% of patients in each vaccine group is much lower when seen as a percentage of total presenting symptoms. The data is summarised in Table 14 and Figures 14.1 and 14.2.

This analysis further emphasises the impact of the MMR and the varicella vaccines on developmental and behavioural problems, and the link between the DPT vaccine and skin and respiratory diseases (especially asthma). The neurological impact of the HPV vaccine is seen clearly, as is the respiratory impact of the Hib vaccine.

Table 14: Comparative Analysis of Disease Groupings (2022)

Symptoms	**DPT**	**MMR**	**Hep B**	**HPV**	**Varic.**	**Hib**	**Mening**	**MMRV**
Developmental / behavioural	**45.3%**	**65.4%**	**42.1%**	**32.3%**	**71.1%**	**42.4%**	**45.5%**	**59.0%**
Neurological	5.9%	5.3%	7.9%	**24.6%**	4.4%	**15.2%**	6.8%	7.7%
Respiratory/ENT	23.3%	12.7%	**23.7%**	6.2%	8.9%	**27.3%**	**22.7%**	12.8%
GIT	8.5%	9.4%	**15.8%**	7.7%	11.1%	3.0%	**13.6%**	10.3%
Skin	**12.9%**	4.7%	5.3%	6.2%	2.2%	9.1%	9.1%	10.3%
Other	4.1%	2.5%	5.3%	**23.1%**	2.2%	3.0%	2.3%	0.0%
Total	**100.0%**	**100.0%**	**100.0%**	**100.0%**	**100.0%**	**100.0%**	**100.0%**	**100.0%**

The additional groupings further emphasise the following two findings:

1. INFANRIX HEXA and Hep B are very similar apart from skin and GIT symptoms, where HEXA is clearly the dominant causative vaccine for skin issues and Hep B for GIT.
2. All vaccines impact the gut - GIT symptoms are significant across every vaccine, but the percentages are consistent, apart from Hib. When looked at as a percentage of participants (rather than of total presenting symptoms), the GIT factor is clearly significant.

Figure 14.1: Comparative Analysis of Disease Groupings (as a percentage of total presenting symptoms) 2022

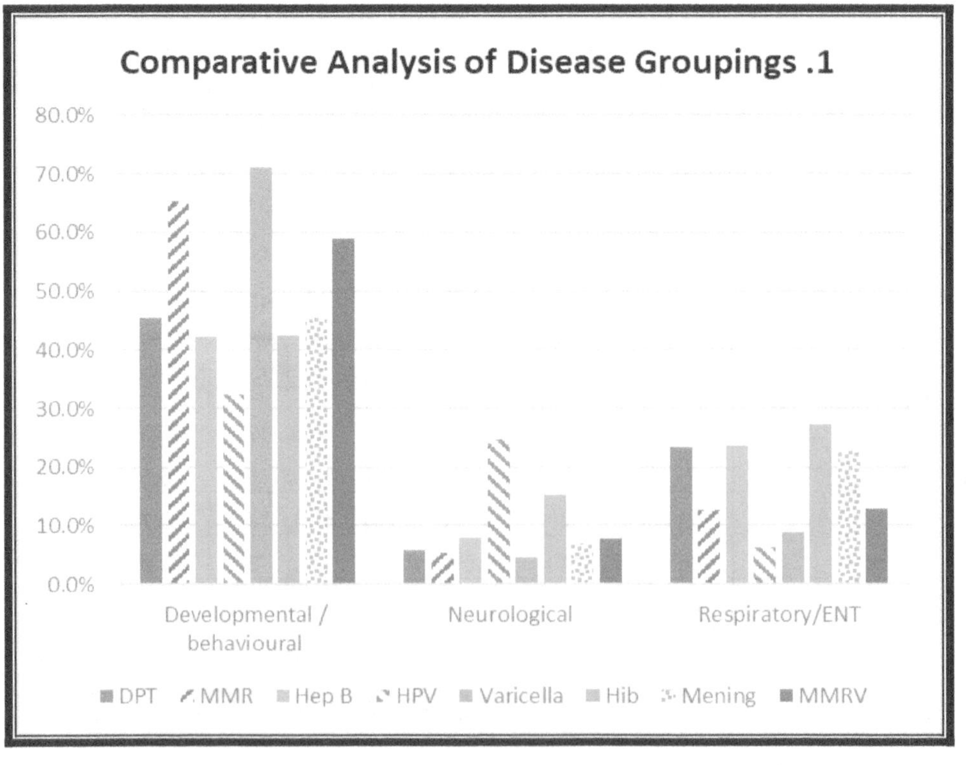

Figure 14.2: Comparative Analysis of Disease Groupings (as a percentage of total presenting symptoms) 2022

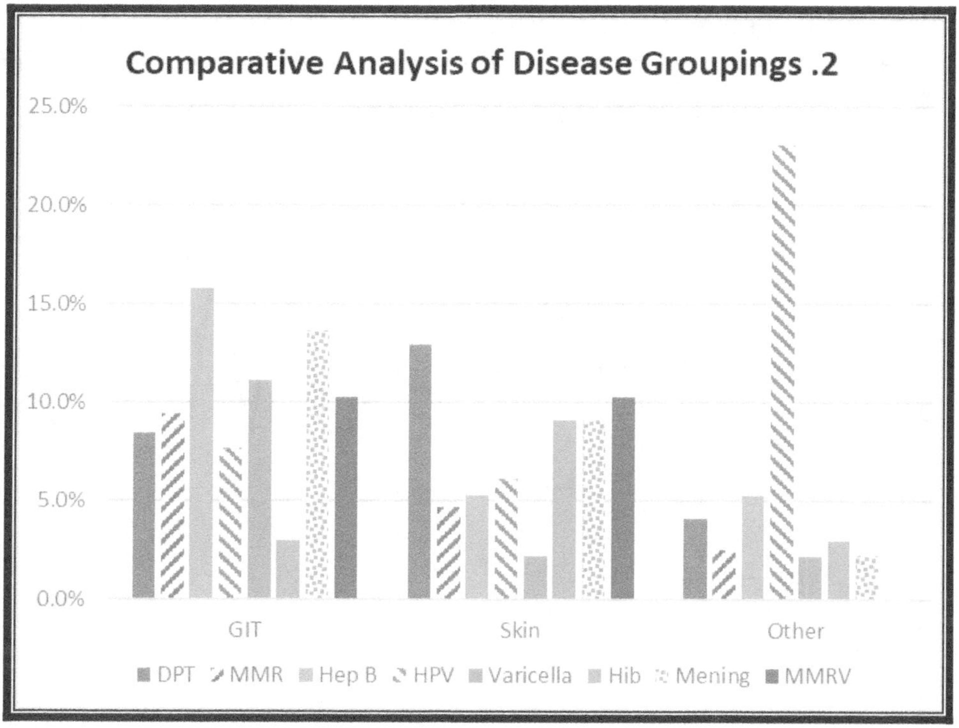

2.10 Symptom Differences Between Males and Females

This is a new section in this 4th edition which was suggested to me by a parent, and I thought it an excellent suggestion to see what the data shows.

Figure 15 speaks for itself, showing that the psychological effect of vaccines on males is significantly greater than for females. This is not surprising given it is known that many more boys are on the spectrum and have aggressive ADHD type symptoms than girls. The physical symptom profiles are similar.

Figure 15: Comparative Symptom Profiles of Males and Females

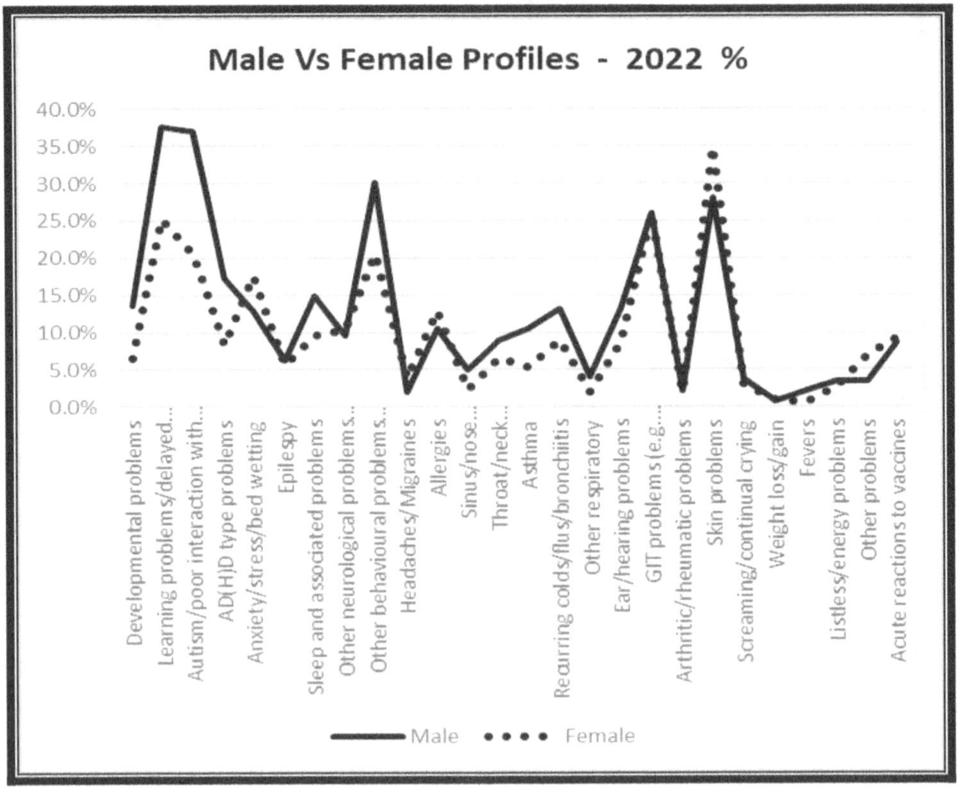

Before moving on to more data analysis, let's look at another case.

2.9 Case 555 – Austin

Overview: I am including this case to show how parents can chose to discontinue treatment when the going gets tough, i.e. when we reach a stage in treatment when the patient hit a layer of cause and reacts to the remedies. In this case there was an immediate and amazing start to the case, and the prognosis was excellent. Early treatment led to clear and significant improvements, but the parents gave up treatment after only seven months, despite such a positive start.

It is of course the parents' choice, and there may be family issues which the practitioner is not aware of – but it can be very disappointing when this happens when the cause of at least some symptoms has been confirmed, and the potential for future improvement appears so great.

29.5.17 1st consultation

Austin Male, DOB 21.2.13

Vaccinated 0, 2, 4, 6, 12, 18 months. Currently at 4 y/o mainstream kinder with an aid.

ASD. Seeing a chiropractor plus has had OT and ST (have now used up allowance)

Observation: was carried into clinic screaming and after 2-3 minutes his father took him outside as he was too distressed. Parents said that this now happens with every appointment and meant that the Speech

Therapists had to discontinue treatment as Austin was unable to participate.

ASD - diagnosed at 3 y/o

Was fine up to 12 months of age.

Straight after the MMR vaccine he stopped eating well (was not fussy eater before this). He lost eye contact for 2 years. Stopped giving or wanting hugs and cuddles. Lost language (he was saying words prior to the vaccine).

He went into his own little world.

NOW: Loves cuddles from parents. Has eye contact with them. Still has no language. No toilet training.

Goes to kinder Mon-Thurs. Is happy to be around the other children but does not play with them. He also loves watching other children on TV.

He seems to get very frustrated now. He can bag his head backwards against a seat if frustrated.

He seems to understand most instructions. He cannot speak so he communicates with his parents by bringing them or their hands to what he wants done.

Has had 2 lots of grommets put into his ears and seemed to improve for a while each time.

Rx. (1) MMR 30 twice weekly, the (2) MMR 200 twice weekly.

29.5.17 Same day of consultation, mother sent following email *"Hello Isaac, thanks for seeing us today. We're shocked and have video footage. It's unbelievable. We just gave him his first dose 30 min ago and then he starts opening cupboards where his trucks and cars are that he hasn't played with in a year. Sitting for 20 min on the floor listening to instructions, like come closer, and is extra happy. He isn't running around. We're freaking out how can anything happen after one dose. Thanks so much. Is this normal, so quick? My husband said if he wasn't here he wouldn't believe it. Thanks. "*

Advised her to wait until repeating the dose.

26.6.17 He is going well.

Rx. Take #2 twice weekly

6.7.19 Some changes

Rx. Give #2 for 2 weeks then #3 MMR M and #4 MMR 10M weekly.

17.7.19 The 2nd week with #2, more settled and eye contact is much better

31.7.19 Going well on #3.

9.8.17 Gave #4 in water. Parents said he was interacting more, but hitting himself,

Rx. keep going with remedies, but come and see me,

25.8.17 2nd consultation

The initial response was very positive. His teachers have noticed a big improvement.

He is noticing other children more. Is more engaged in things. Has fewer outbursts – happier.

His eye contact is much better.

His understanding has improved. He will engage in new activities and understands what he is doing.

He hasn't needed grommets for 6 months now. He will brush his teeth now.
He is less sensory limited. But does have to wear headphones as noise can upset him.
Will do painting and use play dough.

Still is non-verbal – will show parents things.
Food intake is still limited.
Much less head banging, but still happens. Will hit himself now.
Still wants to be on the move.

Rx. #5 MMR 500M then #6 MMR 100M weekly. Takes the doses in water.

5.10.17 He has had an operation. Give #6.

31.10.17 Rx. #7 MMR 500M weekly in water.

14.12.17 Rx. #8 MMR MM, then #9 MMR 10MM fortnightly in water.

19.1.18 Reacted to #8. Started punching, biting, and hitting his head. Told parents to wait, then give one sniff of #8

28.1.18. LAST CONTACT FROM PARENTS. Reported that Austin's sleep is poor. I advised them to see me again to work out what is happeining. They did not come to see me again.

FINAL NOTE: I sent them a letter inviting follow up on 30.12.18, but no response. CASE CLOSED.

2.11 Case and Consultation Profiles

2.11(a) Comparative Analysis of Total and Successful Cases

Figure 15 compares the disease profile of all responses, and successful cases only (whose codes are T1 and T2 in the survey). It indicates that there is little difference between the T1 and T2 profiles, but there is a difference when compared to the profile of all cases.

Figure 15: Comparative Analysis of Total and Successful Cases (2022)

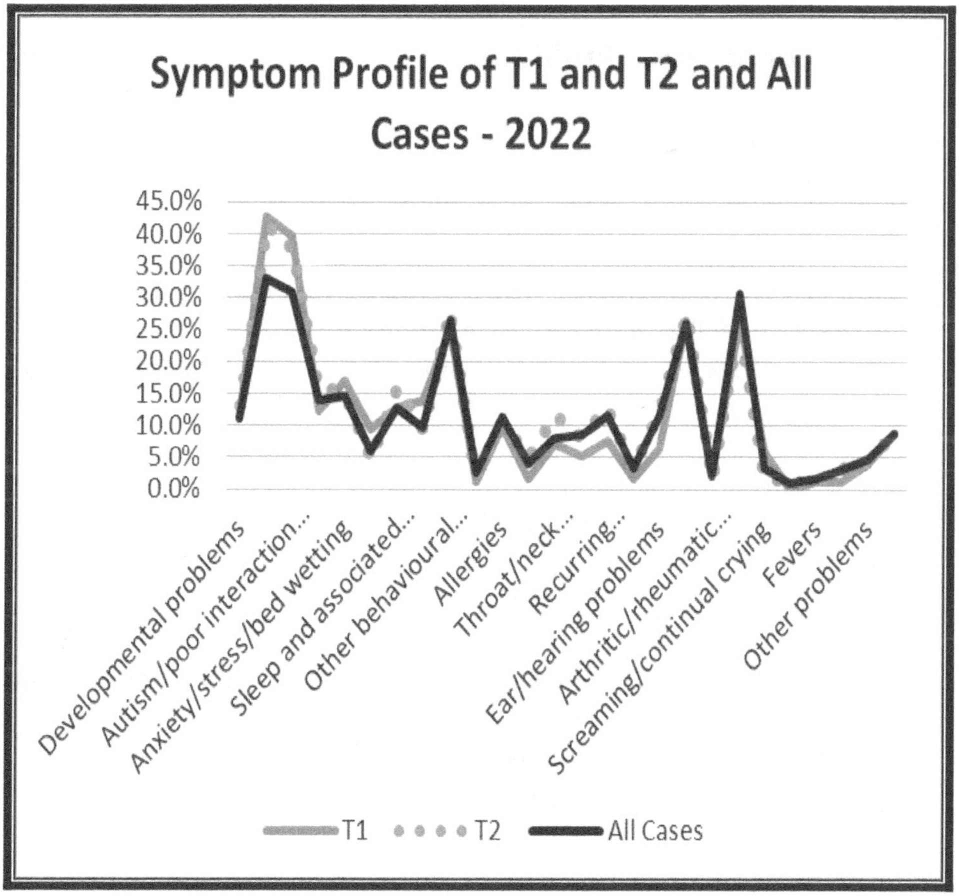

There is a clear difference with the symptom groupings of learning/delayed development and ASD/poor interaction with others. There is a much higher percentage of such cases in the T1/T2 group than for all cases.

This suggests that patients with these symptom groupings respond better to treatment than others. The other symptom profiles are very similar.

2.11(b) Consultation Profile

Table 16 compares the consultation profile of all respondents, successful respondents (T1 and T2), and patients on the autism spectrum.

It shows clearly that patients who attended more consultations (2.29 compared to 1.89) and undertook a greater number of non-consultation follow-ups usually by phone or email (7.12 compared to 5.29) got better results.

This finding is not at all unexpected. It also suggests that both the practitioner and the patients (or their parents) should be aware that the more attention which is given to the case, the more successful the likely outcome.

The figures for patients with a formal diagnosis of autism or who were unambiguously on the spectrum showed the greatest success rate (85.6% after removing non-respondents). There were many more males at 73.2% (an expected result).

A significant difference in figures is the much earlier date when parents first noticed a change in their child (15.5 months for Autism compared to 20.4 and 20.2 months for all cases and T1/T2 cases) compared to the age when the first consultation occurred (75.2, 74.4 and 68.8 months). This is probably due to effect of the first MMR vaccine at 12 months which is certainly a risk factor for autism.

Table 16: Consultation Profile (2022)

Treatment Result/Type (2022)	Total Group	T1 , T2	Autism
#	818 (634 with responses)	429	355 (298 with responses)
All patients T1 , T2 (with resp)	429 (67.7%)		225 (85.6%)
Male (T1, T2)	516 (63.1%)	268 (62.5%)	262 (73.8%)
Female (T1, T2)	302 (36.9%)	161 (37.5%)	93 (26.2%)
* Av. age of first symptoms	20.4 mths	20.2 mths	15.5 mths
* Average age at first consult	74.4 mths	68.8 mths	75.2 mths
Average number of visits	1.89	2.29	2.02
Av. number of contacts	5.29	7.12	6.09

* Note: ages for between 20-30% of respondents were not classified

2.11(c) Successful Consultation Profile

Table 17 shows the percentages of different treatment types within the successful consultations group (T1, T2) and the total group.

Successful treatments were associated with cases where more than one vaccine remedy was used (19.8% to 17.0%). The successful group more often used other remedies as well as the vaccine remedies (60.8% to 55.4%). It should be noted that when I used more than one homoeopathic remedy, it was not mixed with other remedies, and that the different remedies as well as different potencies were spaced apart.

Classical homoeopaths generally prefer to use the fewest number of remedies to achieve a positive result. **This has always been my own preference, but the findings suggest that it is probable I would have helped slightly more patients if I had used remedies covering more than just one vaccine.**

Table 17: Percentage of Successful Consultations (T1, T2) by Treatment Type, Compared with Total Group (2022)

Treatment Type (2022)	T1 , T2		Total Group	
	#	%	#	%
All patients	429		818	
Multiple vaccines implicated	87	20.3	122	14.9
Single vaccines implicated	342	79.7	696	85.1
Multiple vaccine remedies used	85	19.8	139	17.0
Only used vaccine remedies	168	39.2	365	44.6
Vaccine + concurrent rem.	261	60.8	453	55.4

One of the problems with combining the use of different remedies is that one cannot always be certain which remedy did what. However, the careful observation of the timing of remedy reactions will give the practitioner considerable guidance as to the actions of the individual medicines. The most important point is that the patient improves.

It is probable that patients present with several "layers" of problems, and if this is correct then no one single remedy will ever be able to clear all faults. **Vaccines can cause layers due to the shock they impart to a child on all levels.** In such cases no treatment will be totally successful until the vaccine layers are removed.

2.12 Summary of Findings from the Latest Research

2.12.1 Symptom Profiles of Eight Vaccines

(a) **DPT Vaccine (over all periods):** Behavioural problems (ADHD and anger), sleep disorders. General anxiety and learning. SKIN. Asthma and recurring respiratory conditions.

DPT - INFANRIX HEXA Vaccine: BEHAVIOURAL problems (social difficulties, ADHD and anger), sleep disorders. LEARNING delay. General anxiety. SKIN. ALLERGIES. GIT PROBLEMS. Asthma and recurring respiratory conditions.

(b) **MMR Vaccine:** LEARNING, INTERACTIVE (AUTISTIC), GENERAL BEHAVIOURAL ISSUES. GIT PROBLEMS.

Small sample sizes make the following findings suggestive only

(c) **Hep B Vaccines:** SOCIAL INTERACTION AND LEARNING PROBLEMS. General behavioural issues. Allergies. GIT ISSUES. Acute reactions to vaccine.

(d) **HPV (Gardasil) vaccine:** ANXIETY, STRESS. NEUOROLOGICAL PROBLEMS. Headaches. GIT problems. Listless/poor energy.Skin.

(e) **Varicella vaccine:** LEARNING. SOCIAL INTERACTION. General behavioural issues. GIT PROBLEMS.

(f) **Hib Vaccine:** DEVELOPMENTAL AND LEARNING PROBLEMS. ADHD type behaviour. Sleep. Asthma. SKIN.

(g) **Meningococcal vaccine**: Learning. Social interaction problems. General Behavioural Issues. Recurring colds and flu. GIT PROBLEMS. Skin.

(h) **MMRV Vaccine:** LEARNING. SOCIAL INTERACTION (AUTISM). General behavioural problems. GIT and skin issues.

2.12.2 Consultation and Potency Profiles

(a) The more consultations and follow-ups, the greater the likelihood of a successful treatment. This should guide the practitioner and the patient in their approach to treatment of vaccine injured children.

(b) The best results are obtained when more than one vaccine is targeted with remedies, and when other supportive treatment is given.

(c) Higher potencies are needed to get the best results.

2.13 Further Comments

Much more research needs to be undertaken into the possible long-term general health effects of vaccination. As I stated above, it is no credit to orthodox authorities that such work has not been published. The fact that we are looking at conditions that may slowly develop for years after the vaccine has been given, before being diagnosed, means that the task is difficult but not impossible.

The reporting of even immediate adverse events (reactions) from vaccines is extremely lax in Australia. Most doctors simply refuse to acknowledge that vaccines cause injury. The work has been taken up by a parental support group – the Australian Vaccination-Risks Network (AVN). Their excellent work is discussed in Appendix 5.

The research cited above shows that there is evidence of long-term vaccine injury that is presently not acknowledged. This evidence shows that drawing conclusions based only on comparisons of short-term vaccine reactions and possible disease effects is ignoring the largest negative impact of vaccination – the progressive long-term weakening of the overall wellbeing of the recipient.

2.14 Cases: Two "Never Well Since the Vaccine" Cases

2.14.1 Case 245 - "Daniel"

Overview: Daniel's case shows how a situation which began within 20 minutes of vaccination, and continued for 5 months leading to the consultation, can respond to potencies of the vaccine. With hindsight, Daniel would probably have made quicker progress if I had begun with a lower potency of the DPT (to lessen possible reactions) and had given more frequent remedy repetitions.

13.3.90 Daniel was an 11month old child whose mum brought him to see me following a reaction to the third Triple Antigen (DPT) vaccine 5 months earlier, when he was 6 months of age.

She said he was different 20 minutes after the vaccine. That night he wouldn't sleep. His eyes were swollen and glazed the next afternoon. For 6 days he arched his back and screamed. He wouldn't feed properly for 10 days following the vaccine. He would be rigid when picked up. His nappies were like chopped spinach. He lost his smile. He was given homoeopathic Chamomile based on his symptoms.
In all, it took about three weeks to recover from the initial shock of the vaccine.

Daniel has never been well since the vaccine. He has recurring problems with fluid in his ears plus regular ear infections. He is also subject to repeated colds and flu since the vaccine. He developed the flu in November 1989 which lasted until February 1990 when he got a very bad cough where he would hold his breath and feel nauseous at the end of the cough. His mother wondered if it might have been whooping cough.

Rx. (1) DPT 10M, 1 dose weekly. (2) Silica 200, hold until advised.

19.3.90 reacted to DPT 10M – advised to wait.
22.3.90 the reaction has settled, advised to give remedy (2) on 29.3.90.
19.4.90 was better following Silica 200.
5.6.90 has the flu.

22.7.90 (2nd consultation)
Daniel had another hearing test on 10.7.90 which reported mild bilateral hearing loss probably due to fluid in both middle ears. Mother reported that he is better in general since starting the treatment. After the (1) DPT 10M Daniel had a lot of mucus in his throat, now it is much less. He reacted to the remedy, then improved after a few days.

Rx. repeat (1) DPT 10M. New remedy (3) Pulsatilla 3x t.d.s. *(this remedy was given to help drain Daniel's Eustachian tubes).*

12.10.90 Daniel reacted again to (1) DPT 10M for a few days. Appears to be heading towards glue ear.

16.11.90 He is not doing well. Advised to repeat (1) DPT 10M.

23.11.90 His symptoms have cleared up.

6.12.90 He is going well. Advised to repeat (1) DPT 10M on 16.12.90, and get back in touch if there are any problems.

CASE FINISHED

2.14.2 Case 109 – "Jane"

Overview: Jane's case is an example of how inappropriate it is for Government and semi-Government bodies to force people to be vaccinated under threat of failing in studies, of not being employed (such as many nursing students) or being demoted or moved to positions that they do not want, especially when a safe and comparably effective option is available.
The improvement Jane made following the vaccine potency makes it clear that the vaccine was the cause. It also shows how usually effective treatments can be of limited value if the true cause of a problem is not removed. Finally, it shows that conventional medical tests will frequently not show any problems following vaccine injury, despite the obvious fact that the patient is unwell.

15.11.07 I have never met Jane who is 20y/o. Her dad phoned me asking for help, and emailed me on 15.11.07.

Jane had been pressured into having the DTPa vaccine by her University, who threatened her with being failed in a subject she had just successfully studied.

She was vaccinated late afternoon on Thursday 18/10/07. On Saturday 20/10/07 she developed diarrhoea. She came into the family kitchen and collapsed against the fridge, and then to the ground. She breathed with difficulty, was very flushed, had a severe headache, her pulse was 100 and she was faint. She shook, weak muscles, spasms through the neck and back with gagging and stuttering. The injection site was bruised and raised without heat or inflammation.

Her parents took Jane to hospital emergency ward, and she spent the day there with repeated episodes of shaking, stuttering etc about every 15 minutes. The tests conducted by the hospital came back all clear. She was given IV fluids and pain killers, and the hospital doctors said she had a migraine.

Jane had chiropractic treatment on Sunday. The chiropractor also advised rest without stimulation, light, music, sun, tea, coffee, etc. Rest helped her, but by Monday she was worsening again. She visited her GP and had two severe episodes in his clinic. His initial thought was a brain bleed, and Jane was admitted to hospital again for observation and an MRI, which was all clear.

Wednesday 24th she was given a Mora treatment to neutralise the vaccine, and this was repeated 2 weeks later. She took Thuja in potency from 22/10/07 plus vitamin C. She has also had nutritional medicine (her dad is a therapist).

Her dad reported that for the first 10 days following the vaccine Jane spent most of her time in a darkened room alone, resting. After a couple of weeks, she was having only irregular episodes.

However, the day before her father contacted me, Jane had attended University for 2 hours, and then collapsed, with stuttering, loss of muscle strength, and a marked deficit on the left side where she cannot pick up her left foot.

Rx. (1) DPT M as required (single dose, observe reaction, then repeat as symptoms dictate).

6.2.08 Jane is better on the remedy. Rx. DPT 10M.

17.6.08 Jane has greatly improved.
6.8.08 Still better.
Rx. (3) DPT 50M monthly. Take a few monthly doses, then cease when the need for treatment has concluded.
CASE FINISHED

2.15 COVID – Treating "Vaccine" Injury

We live on an amazing and beautiful planet. If the human species were caring, thoughtful, and free of greed, anger and fear we would live in a perfect world. But that is not the case.

In a near-perfect world people like Fauci and Gates and Schwab would be held to account, their assets stripped and used to help the world's most disadvantaged, and their personal freedoms removed by imprisonment for the remainder of their miserable lives.

In a near-perfect world organisations like the CDC and the NIH in the USA, and the NHMRC and TGA in my own country Australia and so many others around the world would be exposed and their leaders sacked, and replaced by real scientists who were independent of the pharmaceutical drug cartels and cared only about the truth.

In a near perfect-world the "experts" who were rolled out by politicians and the media to convince us that the only thing that would save us was vaccination, and social distancing, and masking and lockdowns, and who told us from February 2020 until now that there were no options available other than vaccines and drugs to both prevent and treat SARS-CoV-2, would be publicly exposed as either fools or liars. Fools because they did not know the truth, or liars because they knew the truth but refused to tell us.

And as for politicians and the mainstream media - almost all were worse than useless. Truth avoidance and buck-passing was their way.

There is so much more that can and will be said - but for now I just wish to briefly discuss the treatment of Covid "vaccine" injuries (I use " " as I am not entering into a discussion about genetic engineering and vaccines).

2.15.2 Simple Treatment of Covid "Vaccine" Injuries

Prior to Covid I dealt mainly with vaccine injuries in children who had obvious health issues. Some young women were treated for injuries from the Gardasil vaccine but otherwise I saw very few adults for vaccine injuries.

Since 2020 things have changed. Many parents of apparently healthy children are getting them a basic vaccine detox using homeopathic potencies of the different childhood vaccines. My early data shows that about one third of these patients react to the vaccine potencies which means that the vaccine IS still causing them harm in an unrecognised way. And we treat that injury.

But now I am seeing many (mainly) adults who are suffering from long-term effects from the different Covid "vaccines" - in homeopathy we call this a "never-well-since" state, and it is a crucial point in any case taking.

My general approach is to begin with using potencies of the specific vaccine which began the "never-well-since" state. At times I use potencies of the Spike Protein.

Related through the Spike Protein are a noticeable minority of people with long-Covid, i.e. never well since a SARS-CoV-2 infection. The use of SARS-CoV-2 Nosodes and potencies of the Spike Protein have proved simple and useful.

My latest data is shown in Tables 18.1 and 18.2. **This is very much work in progress as seen by the large percentage of T6 classifications in Table 18.1 – no follow-up.** Many of these people were not due to provide a follow-up because they just began treatment in August and September 2023. Others just simply did not provide a follow-up. This classification is removed in Table 18.2 as well as those who simply chose not to take the remedies provided.

Some may think that people didn't respond because the remedies either didn't work, or made the person worse, but long experience with chasing up potential respondents shows that this is not the case.

Table 18.1: Latest Clinical Data – 2023 %

	Treatment		Basic
	CVvax Injury	Long Covid	Vaxxed Detox
T1 – Strong imp/ment	23.7	37.5	6.1
T2 - Improvement	8.5	23.2	2.6
T3 - No improvement	3.4	0.0	0.0
T4 - Worse	0.0	0.0	0.0
T5 - Unclear + and -	2.5	3.6	0.0
T6 - No follow up	50.8	25.0	61.4
T7 – React + no f/up	0.0	0.0	0.0
No reaction (T3)	5.1	-	14.9
Not taken	1.7	7.1	2.6
Worse, then stop (T3)	0.8	3.6	0.0
Reactions (T5)	3.4	-	12.3
Total	100.0	100.0	100.0

Experience shows that many who do not respond achieved what they needed and moved on, ignoring requests to advise progress.
So, Table 18.2 provides a potentially more useful indication of the value of the remedies. And it must be read carefully.

Each column looks at a different aspect of therapy.

(1) The treatment of injuries for Covid "vaccines": 67.9% of respondents reported improvements.
(2) Treatment of "long Covid": 89.5% of respondents reported improvements.
(3) Basic vaccine detox in apparently healthy children: 41.5% of respondents reported no reaction to the remedies given (suggesting the vaccines had not led to long-term injury). 58.5% reported a reaction, of which 24.4% reported an improvement and 34.1% are still undergoing treatment. **This means that the majority of apparently healthy children were vaccine injured.**

Table 18.2: Latest Clinical Data, Excluding T6 and "Not Taken" - %

	Treatment		Basic
	CVvax Injury	Long Covid	Vaxxed Detox
T1 – Strong imp/ment	50.0	55.3	17.1
T2 - Improvement	17.9	34.2	7.3
T3 - No improvement	7.1	0.0	0.0
T4 - Worse	0.0	0.0	0.0
T5 - Unclear + and -	5.4	5.3	0.0
T7 – React + no f/up	0.0	0.7	0.0
No reaction (T3)	10.7	-	41.5
Worse, then stop (T3)	1.8	5.3	0.0
Reactions (T5)	7.1	-	34.1
Total	100.0	100.0	100.0

PART 3: Conclusions

Question 3: How Can We Prevent Vaccine Injury?

3.1 Prevention of Vaccine Injury

The only certain way to prevent vaccine injury is - don't be vaccinated.

Some homoeopaths recommend a variety of procedures prior to vaccination to minimise the likelihood of vaccine injury, including:

(i) Taking potencies of the relevant vaccines before vaccination
(ii) Taking the nosodes of the relevant diseases before vaccination
(iii) Taking Thuja (or other anti-vaccination remedies) in high potency before vaccination
(iv) Obtaining constitutional treatment before vaccination

I would certainly support the constitutional option as being worthwhile at any time. The more energetically stronger a person is before receiving a toxic shock to the system, which is what vaccination is, the more likely that they will survive unharmed, i.e. the stronger the *life force,* the greater the chance of it correcting imbalances caused by the vaccine.

There is no doubt that homoeopathic anti-miasmic treatment, good diet and lifestyle, appropriate use of other modalities, etc will also help to maximise health and lessen the potential for vaccine injury.

However, it is my experience that nothing can guarantee the prevention of vaccine injury except not being vaccinated.

Some homoeopaths believe that vaccine injury can be prevented by giving potencies of vaccines, or other remedies such as Thuja, before vaccination. I don't believe that we can make such guarantees given that there is no published data that I am aware of clearly demonstrating a protective effect. I know of colleagues that I respect who make claims of protection, but I am not comfortable doing this without evidence.

I am supported in this view by Dr Tinus Smits, who states that "Homoeopaths used to recommend, and sometimes still do, Thuja 30C before vaccination. Personally, I have had unfortunate experiences with this and have never been able to confirm its efficacy."

However, Dr Smits routinely supports option (i) above to minimise the likelihood of vaccine injury. He gives a dose of the intended vaccine in 200c potency, two days before the vaccine and again on the same day the vaccine is given. He then gives the remedy a month later in 30c, 200c, M and 10M potencies over some weeks (see Appendix 2).

But the only certain way to prevent vaccine injury is don't be vaccinated.

I recommend to parents who are choosing to vaccinate their child, to give large doses of Vitamin C a week before and a week after the vaccine. The purpose is to minimise the risk of toxic shock from the vaccines. It was an idea suggested to me by the late Dr Glenn Dettman many years ago, following his pioneering work with Dr Archie Kalokerionos in the 1970's and beyond.
Kalokerinos A (1974) *Every Second Child.* Thomas Nelson Ltd., Australia

I also recommend giving the child age-appropriate probiotics and Omega supplements for 10 days before and after each vaccine. But there is **no guarantee** that these will work to prevent vaccine injury

If you must vaccinate your child, then the recommendations from Swiss homoeopath Dr Elmiger, summarised by Dr Smits, make a lot of sense.

a. Delay giving vaccines until the child is older, 10-12 months; (2 months is far too young).
b. Don't give multiple vaccines at the one time (one vaccine needle only). NOTE: this does not mean splitting say a 4 valent vaccine (covering 4 diseases) into 4 needles with one antigen only for the simple reason that this would mean 4 times more aluminium, 4 times more formaldehyde, etc.
c. Don't give vaccines so close to each other (two months apart is too frequent).
d. Don't give vaccines for as many diseases (cover only potentially serious diseases).
e. Don't give the next vaccines until a child has recovered from the previous vaccines.
f. Treat any immediate vaccine injury.
g. Never vaccinate a child who is ill or not fully recovered from an acute disease.

As comprehensive as these recommendations are, the most common form of vaccine injury is long-term injury which may not manifest for months and often years following the vaccine. So, the fact that a patient has been vaccinated with no obvious immediate complications is not sufficient to ensure point (g) is met, and therefore the success of this approach may be compromised.

The only certain way to prevent vaccine injury is - don't be vaccinated.

The use of homoeopathic immunisation (***homœoprophylaxis***) allows parents to choose a form of immunisation that is comparably effective to vaccination, but without the risk of toxic or dynamic injury. The most comprehensive publication on this topic is my book *The Complete Practitioners Manual of Homœoprophylaxis.* The 7th edition of my book *Vaccination & Homœoprophylaxis? A Review of Risks and Alternatives.* Is helpful for parents who are new to the issue of vaccine injury.

The former is designed for practitioners wanting to give HP to their patients. The latter is a comprehensive resource for parents who want options, and for practitioners who may be unfamiliar with this aspect of the homoeopathic method.

They squarely address the issues of safety and effectiveness of both vaccination and homœoprophylaxis. Both books include the latest research from Cuba where over 9.8 million people have been homeopathically immunised against swine flu against swine flu in 2010.

Being a more recent book, *The Complete Practitioners Manual of Homœoprophylaxis* gives even more up to date data. It focuses just on HP (not vaccines) and provides practitioners and parents with a template of a homeopathic immunisation program I use in Australia, as well as discussing overseas travel options in detail.

What our data shows is that parents can avoid the risk of vaccine injury if they wish, but still ensure that their child has a significant level of protection against potentially serious infectious diseases.

Orthodox people will claim there is no evidence to support the safety and effectiveness of this method which was first used in 1799 (vaccination first used in 1796).

However, two articles I published in 2019 quantified the use of homœoprophylaxis in 3 countries in over 250 million people on an annualised basis.

The original article are:
Golden I. Large Homœoprophylaxis: Brief and Long-Term Interventions**.** *American Journal of Homeopathic Medicine*. Winter, **2019; 112**(1): 31-36.

Golden I. Large Homœoprophylaxis Interventions by Government Institutions. *Similia*. **2019**; **31**(2):14-19.

A reworking of these articles is freely available at the following address:

Golden I. The Potential Value of Homœoprophylaxis in Endemic and Epidemic Conditions. Homeopathy 360. 1.4.2019. https://homeopathy360.com/2019/04/01/the-potential-value-of-homoeoprophylaxis-in-endemic-and-epidemic-conditions/

Most of the interventions were carried out by government authorities or government accredited institutions.

We have a LOT of evidence.

3.2 Cases: Two Cases of "Epilepsy with the Lot"

3.3 Case 86 - "Jenny"

Overview: Jenny's case is a special one for me, because it was the first time that I saw such a dramatic positive response to a range of potencies of the suspected vaccine, and how this type of treatment could literally turn a person's life around. Jenny had been brought in by her mum. She hardly spoke, and was living a sheltered and incomplete life. A little over a year later she was outgoing, happy, fully functioning, and engaged to be married. Of course, no one can say what her life would have been 16 years later (as I write this book), but personally I have no doubt that the vaccine potencies helped Jenny to lead a "normal" life.

I saw Jenny for the first time in January 1991 – she was 18 years old. She was brought in by her mum who did most of the talking. Jenny sat quietly in the office with her head down.

She was diagnosed as being epileptic and was taking significant amounts of Epilim and Tegratol daily. She had been on medication since she was 8 years old, but still has turns, and they are getting worse.

ATTACKS: She knows they are coming. Just before a turn she feels panicky. They last 1-2 minutes. She will call out. Her eyes open, and stare, then hands go stiff and spastic. Grates teeth and dribbles, purses lips. Can be aggressive during turns. Cannot talk after the turn even if she tries hard to.

Six months ago, she had dental work involving amalgam and had a serious reaction.

Her mum said Jenny has seen a lot of doctors. She now spends a lot of time sleeping. She has regular nausea and vomiting which is aggravated by the medication. Regularly has a stale taste in her mouth.

When she was 18 months of age, she reacted to the triple action vaccine, including several convulsions. Since then, she was prone to catching regular childhood diseases.

At 8 years of age, she had a turn and was diagnosed as being epileptic. It was a time of great stress, she was having dental work, and he parents had separated.

From 10-13 years she had kidney infections, plus recurring bowel problems with alternating diarrhoea and constipation.

She struggled academically at high school. Passed year 10 in Queensland. Had difficulty finding work, and is presently working in a laundry.

24.1.91 Rx (1) DPT M take one dose.
Was also given (2) Amalgum 200 with instructions to take one dose when directed.

1.2.91 Mother phoned. Nausea and vertigo have reduced. Has had fewer attacks. Is feeling much better in general. They decided to reduce the Epilim (despite my instructions not to). Told to repeat (1) as needed.

10.5.91 Came for second consultation. Things were going very well taking remedy (1) weekly, until she ran out a month ago. Since then she has become more unwell.

One thing that was obvious to me was the change in Jenny. She was bright and bubbly, looked me in the eye, and this time she did most of the talking.

Rx (3) DPT 10M, but instructed to keep on (1) until told to change to (3). *(note: the reason for this was that I felt the M potency was still active, and should not be changed until it had done all it was capable of).*

16.5.91 Phoned. Starting to feel good again. She had three doses of (1).

6.6.91 Hs been taking (1) every second day. Is still having problems with her pharmaceutical medication which causes nausea and dizziness. She must keep her head very still when walking. However, is still feeling much better in general.

6.7.91 Phoned. Has been taking (1) daily, and has not had any turns. Is feeling really well.

12.8.91 Third consultation. Has been taking (3) daily. Started to get turns again when reduced (1) to every 2-3 days, but since taking (3) has been much better again. Has reduced medication even further. Energy much better.

12.3.92 Fourth and final consultation. Going very well. Is yawning more lately.

Rx. (4) DPT 50M to take as needed.

Final note. The last time I heard from Jenny was a call to advise that she had become engaged. She was completely off Epilim and on a minimal dose of Tagratol (which she and her mum had managed).

She had gone from being an introverted, tired, unwell person who struggled with life, to being a vibrant young woman ready to start a new life.
The remedy which assisted Jenny was ascending potencies of the triple antigen vaccine (DPT). The remedy would not have helped her unless the vaccine had been the cause of her "epilepsy".

CASE FINISHED

3.4 Case 5 - "Kylie"

Overview: Kylie's case is one of many cases of a patient developing seizures and being diagnosed as being epileptic following vaccination. It also shows how potencies of the suspect vaccine can make a great difference. Some readers may wonder why I am including a case of a mature woman in a book on vaccine injured kids. The answer is that Kylie was injured as a child, and the injury had lasted well into adulthood.

8.8.2000 1st consultation.

Kylie was a 31 year old single woman when she presented. She was receiving the invalid pension due to her condition.

She had been a healthy child. She had been bottled fed, was quiet, happy, smiled a lot, didn't grizzle. One day she simply collapsed. It seemed like a minor incident. Then a month later she collapsed again, convulsed, frothed at the mouth with staring eyes. At 18 months of age she was diagnosed as epileptic and she has been on medication from then, and was currently on Epilim 700 twice daily. Ever since the first attack she experienced problems with her gums and teeth, and has dribbled ever since then.

Now, her grand mal seizures are controlled by the medication, but she experiences small seizures a few times each week. They are worse from emotions, stress, wanting to please, and pre-menstrually. Her hands will shake, her eyes stare, and she dribbles. She will sit down for a few minutes, then she will come out of it.

She can suffer from pre-menstrual migraines, which can also trigger a fit. She clenches her feet and toes a lot.

Now, she described herself as an outgoing, very friendly person. She can be very talkative with people she knows, although is more quiet at home. She can be a bit lonely, wanting the company of people her own age. She is very lacking in self confidence, and finds making decisions difficult. She dropped out of school after year 10 after experiencing difficulty keeping up at school. She is on an invalid pension but does volunteer work at kindergartens. Little children love her, and will go up to her readily.

She can also be very determined and stubborn. Occasionally she will get angry quickly if her mind is made up, then can be apologetic later. She likes to follow a routine (she double checks that doors are locked). She normally has a lot of patience with cross stitching and will spend hours doing it.

She wears a hearing aid, and doesn't hear all the time
She enjoys cold weather. Hot weather will aggravate all her symptoms.

Rx. (1) Baryta Sulph 200 weekly *(I began with a possible "constitutional" remedy)*

15.8.2000 gave Kylie (2) DPT M, one dose every 2 weeks.

26.9.2000 (2nd consultation)
The number of minor fits has reduced, although she had a very bad headache pre-menstrually, then had a minor fit.
Her energy has not been so good, but then a relative came to visit with a 1 year old child, and Kylie has been upset by this.

Rx. (1) Baryta Sulph 200 weekly, (3) DPT 10M every 2 weeks. Do not take remedies on the same day.

6.2.2001 (3rd consultation)
Has been really good. "I feel happy, the best I have been for many years".
Still is taking (1) and (3) as directed. Takes an extra dose of (3) if she has a migraine, and it helps prevent a fit.
She has been on a candida diet through an orthomolecular GP
However, her hearing is bad. The doctor says her ears are full of wax.

Rx. (4) DPT 50M every 3 weeks, alternating with (5) Baryta Sulph M every 3 weeks. *(Note made to consider the remedy Bufo next if required).*

7.9.2001 (4th consultation)
NO MORE FITS.
Still has problems with her ears and hearing.
Has been feeling a bit lonely lately. Her mum is trying to help by getting her to mix with others her own age.

Rx. (6) DPT 100M monthly. (7) Pulsatilla 6, one or two doses daily *(the Pulsatilla is given to help drain the ears).*

CASE FINISHED

I have since wondered on many occasions whether many children who are diagnosed as being epileptic are in fact vaccine injured, and whether appropriate treatment for vaccine injury at the time would prevent the need for years of epileptic drugs with their consequent side-effects.

Personally, I never classify patients with a similar case history of being free of seizures prior to vaccination as being "epileptic", but simply as being vaccine injured. Just imagine how different the practice of orthodox medicine would be if all doctors took the same view!

Question 4: How Do We Treat Vaccine Injury?

4.1 Treatment of Vaccine Injury

By the time that Compton Burnett published his famous little work *Vaccinosis – and its Cure by Thuja* in 1884, homoeopaths knew that vaccination was potentially dangerous. One unintended consequence of Burnett's work is that it influenced recent generations of homoeopaths to believe that Thuja was an effective antidote against all vaccines, when in fact it is only useful against smallpox vaccination (which ceased being administered many years ago), or for those few patients whose constitutional remedy is "similar" to Thuja.

My approach is generally conservative. If the injury is recent, I usually begin with a single dose of the suspect vaccine in a 30c or a 200c potency and observe for one or two weeks. This ensures that healing reactions in any highly sensitive or unstable patients will be minimised, and certainly will be able to be recognised before any further doses are given. I have also treated some patients using a series of potencies (e.g. 30, 200, M, 10M) to test Dr Smit's approach.

If the vaccine was given many years before (remembering that many adult patients are still injured from vaccines given maybe 30+ years earlier), and the patient appears reasonably robust, I may begin with a single dose of an M (= 1,000c) or a 10M potency, once again observing for a few weeks before making a decision as to remedy repetition or an increase in potency. I will then slowly work up potencies of the vaccine for as long as results are obtained. I have not infrequently given 100M and MM potencies.

In some cases, the vaccine potency alone gives remarkable results, however I have preferred to combine this treatment with constitutional treatment if the patient agrees (some are happy with initial results and don't follow up over time). I believe this gives the patient the best possibility of restoring their health to the highest possible level.

It is also possible to treat the aetiological "layer" caused by vaccination with remedies other than vaccine potencies. Kent listed 9 remedies in his repertory under the rubric "vaccination", and van Zandvoort's RUV lists at least 51 remedies. I repeat again, Thuja is usually not the appropriate remedy to treat vaccine injury; it is just one of many possible "similars".

Readers can see that a variety of approaches are possible. This shows that we have tremendous flexibility within the Law/Principle of Similars. The use of vaccine potencies to treat vaccine injury is a practical use of the aetiological similimum, one of four possible similimums within the Law/Principle of Similars.
Golden I (2006) Homoeopaths and the Law of Similars. *Similia*, Vol. 18, No.2, December. Pages 3-7.

Differences in treatment don't mean that one practitioner is correct, and the other incorrect, but that a variety of treatment methods are possible, especially if we carefully respond to the reactions and subsequent symptom changes of our patients. I believe this gives the patient the best possibility of restoring their health.

The late Dr Tinus Smits from the Netherlands undertook pioneering work with vaccine injured children. His recommendations are shown in Appendix 3. He recommended the following treatment protocol:

To treat chronic PVS is to administer the potentised vaccine at four different potencies on four consecutive days; the first day 30C, the second day 200C, the third day 1M and the fourth day 10M. In each case about 10 globules should be dissolved in the (dry) mouth. Do not eat or drink or brush the teeth for half an hour before or after this administration to allow the medicament to act without interference.

If the symptoms are aggravated after one of the four potencies it is always necessary to wait until the reaction is over before continuing treatment. In such cases the same potency is then repeated. This procedure is continued as long as necessary for the patient's reaction to cease, normally after one or two repeat doses. The series is then completed. It is also possible to treat a severe reaction with a solution of the 30C. For this, ten globules are dissolved in half a glass of water which is administered, a sip or teaspoonful at a time, for one or two days. The most common reaction is fever, which does not require further treatment. If the child is vulnerable, as for example as a result of serious vaccine-related complications or if oversensitivity is anticipated, each potency can be administered weekly. Severe reactions can similarly be treated by weekly repeats of the same potency until no reaction is clearly discernible. If the disorder has not completely cleared up after three weeks, the whole series can be repeated. One to three series is usually sufficient.

In acute cases the treatment is largely similar, differing only in that the preference in acute cases is given to aqueous solutions of a 30C or 200C as described above. This solution is administered at the rate of a sip or a teaspoonful an hour for a number of days; three doses are usually sufficient. See case 6, Ragma.

Even where the post-vaccination syndrome is of several years' standing it can still be treated successfully, as is shown by case 7, where the patient had suffered for eleven years, and case 8; with a prehistory of 17 years. In both cases the complaints were effectively fully cured.

See www.post-vaccination-syndrome,com/3890/treatment.aspx (accessed 16.7.19).

I fully support Dr Smits formal protocol and use it at times. As I said earlier, there is no one single correct method. I have no doubt that in many cases different approaches would probably yield similar results.

The reason for this is simple. Homoeopathic remedies do not heal the patient. **They remove blockages and injury that prevent the body's own self-healing mechanism from healing.** We have within us the capacity to heal. What we must do is remove recurring obstacles to cure in our daily lives and remove the fundamental chronic causes of our ill health, one of which may be vaccine injury.

If the remedies can remove a layer of injury, the self-healing mechanism WILL work to its best ability to partially heal. There is rarely only one chronic problem, so one line of treatment will need to be followed up with appropriate treatment of other chronic issues (including the chronic miasms which most homoeopaths believe are the root causes of chronic illness).

So whether vaccine injury is removed by a series of single doses or by a number of doses given in quick succession, whether only one potency is used or whether a number of potencies are used, the end result of successful treatment is the same – the self-healing mechanism will begin to work more effectively.

That is the true purpose of our treatment.

4.2 More Case Studies

I would like to share some more cases with you, both successful and unsuccessful. The case numbers are just an internal numbering system and have no other significance. Real names are not used. The full case notes are not given to make for easier reading. In homoeopathy, the patients' words are important, so the notes tend to be in plain English, which has not been "doctored".

I will begin with an immediate adverse reaction to the Gardasil vaccine.

4.3 Case 134 - "Jessica"

Overview: Jessica's case is very instructive in demonstrating how few doctors in Australia are prepared to acknowledge vaccine injury, even when the facts are unambiguous. Such an attitude is of course not only unscientific, it is fundamentally dishonest. This case also shows how symptomatic treatment is often helpful, but not sufficient to finish off a case when the true cause of the disturbance has not been treated.

6.3.08 - 10.10am Jessica had 1st HPV injection in her left arm, and was put into a room for observation. She had minor shakes, then went back to her class. Her friends noticed tremors and insisted that she went to the school sick bay. She also developed a headache and nausea.
11.02am school phoned mother to advise that Jessica had an adverse reaction to the vaccines and needed to be taken home.
11.30am mother signed Jessica out of school, and her hands were shaking uncontrollably, and she was feeling nauseous.

2pm Jessica saw a nurse at a medical clinic, who got a GP to examine her. The GP said he had never seen a reaction to a vaccine like this before. He phoned the Children's Immunisation Clinic who said the symptoms were a reaction to the stress of having a needle, and not because of the vaccine itself. Jessica's mother was advised that the problem should not get worse overnight, but to bring her back if it did.

Later that day, Jessica's legs began shaking uncontrollably, and her body was almost convulsing. Jessica's parents took her to the local hospital at 6.40pm, who told them to give Jessica Panadol, and that reactions to vaccines occur within 15 minutes of the vaccines being administered.

10pm went back to the hospital as the shaking kept getting worse. A doctor eventually saw her and prescribed Diazepan and Panadol which were administered at 11.15pm. Home at 12.35 am

11.3.08 Jessica was brought for treatment by her parents. Her hands and legs were still shaking. She was anxious about her health because of the shaking.

Rx. Jessica was given 3 remedies. (1) Thuja 200 *(the only remedy with the rubric – shaking of extremities following vaccination),* (2) HPV 200, and (3) DPT M (the potency of the HPV vaccine was not available at that time, and the DPT vaccine contained some of the chemicals in the HPV vaccine).

17.3.08 Some improvement, followed by a worsening, gave (4) Thuja M, t.d.s.

4.4.08 (4) Thuja M had reduced the trembling. Ran out a week ago, and steadily worsened. Also complained of pains in her chest for 5-10 minutes. Rx (5) Thuja 10M b.d.

4.5.08 finally obtained a 200c potency of the Gardasil vaccine and posted to Jessica.

Rx. (6) Gardasil 200. Take one dose and report.

16.5.08, (6) Gardasil 200 reduced the shaking, but she has developed some burning in her knees.

23.5.08. Significant improvement. Very occasional "shivers" lasting about half a minute, plus a buzzing feeling in her left shoulder.
30.5.08 Had a good week. Shivers down body. Give a triple dose.
16.6.08. Triple dose stopped tremors.

CASE FINISHED

The next two cases, 101 and 207, are included to emphasise to parents the real need to keep going until cases are finished, that is until the causes of the child's symptoms have been fully dealt with. In both cases improvements were made, but almost certainly greater improvements would have been possible with continued treatment.

4.4 Case 101 – "Billy"

Overview: Billy's case is an example of working with a vaccine potency (to treat the cause) and an intercurrent symptomatic remedy (to treat manifesting symptoms). This case progressed well, but the parents ceased to follow up. Interestingly, the second consultation occurred because Billy told his mother it was time to see me again. He obviously noted the changes caused by the treatment. I would have expected to work up potencies of the DPT vaccine until they were no longer effective, or until a different symptom picture emerges.

Billy was over 7 years old when I saw him on 30.10.07.
His mum said that she brought Billy to see me because of behavioural problems – it was hard to get him to agree to anything at home. His concentration was very poor, and he would rarely finish his work. He was overactive.

She also said that he was impulsive and very aggressive. Billy said he didn't know why. He won't play with other children – he will walk up to them and push them. He finds it very hard to interact with them. As a consequence, lots of children are afraid of Billy because they don't know what he will do next.

His mum said that Billy had been unsettled from about 6-8 months of age, when he was sickly and grizzly. She believed it was from teething. Billy has always ground his teeth.

Physically, he has had problems with chronic sinus congestion from 1½ years of age. It varies now, but his voice is always hoarse. It is worse on rising when Billy can hardly speak. His tonsils and adenoids were removed earlier this year. He has been a mouth breather for many years.

Rx. Alternate (1) DPT M and (2) Stramonium M fortnightly until response

15.11.07 Mother phoned to say that Billy was more aggressive after both remedies.

I then did not hear from Billy's mother again until 6.6.08 after contacting her by mail inquiring after Billy's progress. She told me that she had kept giving Billy the remedies periodically, and he has made slow but steady progress. She said that friends and family have commented on his progress. He is less erratic and not as hyperactive. However, he is still not right.
6.6.08 Rx. Give Billy a triple dose of (1) DPT M

20.6.08 Mother reported that Billy was very good after the triple dose, but the effect has started to wear off.
Rx. (3) DPT 10M

12.7.08 Better on (3).

13.8.08 Slipping back – told mother that it was time to see me again.

1.9.08 (2nd consultation).
Mother said Billy had improved dramatically up to late July, then slipped back late August. July and August were big months and possibly unsettling. However, in general is still going well.

Rx. (4) DPT 50M, (5) DPT 100M - begin with (4), and take doses only as needed.

No further feedback from parents. CASE CLOSED.

4.5 Case 207 – "Sally"

Overview: Sally's case is one where more work could have been done, but because she was so much better, treatment was not continued by the parents. It was a very good sign homoeopathically that she finished with a return of a skin eruption (even though it was not mentioned in the consultation). The Laws of Nature dictate that healing must occur from within out – so the skin should be the last to heal, as it was in Sally's case.

13.5.96 1st consultation

Sally was 1½ years old when her parents brought her in. She was thin and pale in appearance.

She was prone to recurring colds from 4 months of age, and ear problems since 12 months of age. Grommets were inserted in February 1996, which had help to improve fluid build-up behind both ears. Her sleep had improved and she cried less.

She had a bad ear infection 2 weeks earlier and was prescribed 3 courses of antibiotics. This was preceded by recurring colds.

Sally was vaccinated at 3 months of age and 6 months of age, and nothing since then.

She was breastfed for 12 months of age. Crawled 7-8 months, walked at 11 months, first teethed at 9 months of age.

Sally has been happier since the grommets. She likes her mother's attention.

She is aggressive to children her own age and smaller (she will pull their hair out). She takes time to feel relaxed with new adults but is not shy at all with older children. She wants what other children are playing with and is possessive with her own toys.

If upset, she weeps and seeks consolation. She will bang her head on the floor or the window if she cannot get her own way.

Her parents' health is good, as it that of her siblings.

Rx. Begin with (1) Pulsatilla 30 twice daily as an ear drainage remedy. Then alternate (2) DPT M and (3) Bacillinum 200 every 2 weeks unless reaction. The last remedy is often helpful when there is a recurring pattern of respiratory infections.

21.5.96. Mother phoned. Didn't feel much benefit from the Pulsatilla 30. Gave (2) DPT M then 4 days later Sally developed a runny nose, and was sleeping better.

15.7.96 Two months later, Sally came again. She has been taking (2) DPT M regularly. Her ears have been very good, and she is much better within herself. Lately has developed eczema on her legs, with some itching on her stomach and behind her knees.

Rx DPT 10M every two weeks as needed.

CASE FINISHED

4.6 Case 90 – "Teddy"

Overview: Teddy's case shows a common pattern of skin eruptions with respiratory symptoms. The case was significantly improved with potencies of the MMR vaccine. A potency of the DPT vaccine was given at the end to clear likely injury, but there was no follow up.

23.2.04 1st consultation.

Teddy was nearly 2 years of age when his mum brought him to see me. She said he had been teething on and off for 12 months. When it is difficult his sleep pattern becomes bad, he dribbles, he experiences a lot of pain, and he often gets a cold.

His first significant problem was eczema in the folds of his elbows, and for the last 12 months on his legs, especially the shins and calves. Itching was aggravated by warmth, including the warmth of bed.

His second significant problem was recurring colds. He had croup at 9 months of age, and it has recurred from time to time. He still has some wheezing.

Teddy's milestones were unusual. He talked early but didn't crawl until 10 months, and didn't walk until 18 months. He began teething at 5 months of age. Teething has been very difficult over his life.

His mother described Teddy as a placid child, gentle, easy going (his sister wants to be in control, and he doesn't mind). He is very affectionate. He doesn't cry easily. He gets on well with other children. He is very attached to his mother. His mother describes Teddy as a "reasonable" person.

He is very interested in mechanical things. He loves the farm. Fearless – is good in new situations. Is OK meeting new people.

He is generally a warm person.
Loves chocolate, but it aggravates his skin. Likes fruit but not veggies. Likes carbohydrate foods.

His mother had eczema, asthma and hay fever, and his maternal grandfather had asthma.

Rx. (1) MMR 10M monthly, alternated with (2) Calc Phos M monthly. *(note that the MMR vaccine was given due to the timing of the worsening of his symptoms around the vaccine, and the Calc Phos because I felt it suited Teddy on a constitutional and miasmic level).*

10.5.04 (2nd consultation)
He reacts when he has either remedy – is tired and grumpy for a few days. The eczema on his legs has improved by 40-50%. Croup possibly worse in the colder weather of winter.

Rx. (1) MMR 10M monthly, alternating with (4) Calc Phos 10M. (3) Hepar Sulph 200 as needed acutely for croup like symptoms.

9.8.04 (3rd consultation)
Teddy is progressing well. He is not as grumpy after each dose of (1) and (4) now. He is having soy and no cheese (the eczema and mucus or conjunctivitis will aggravate if he eats the wrong foods, especially dairy foods).
He has only had one attack of croup (last winter was having attacks almost weekly). Has only had 1 cold this winter. Also, no signs of asthma.

Rx. (4) Calc Phos 10M, alternating with (5) MMR 50M monthly.

13.2.06 (4th consultation)
Teddy's immune system is now much better. His eczema is much better, and the cycle of colds has been broken.

Rx. (5) DPT 10M every 3 weeks. *(the symptoms suggested that the MMR potencies had done their job, and the DPT was given to remove any residual injury from that vaccine).*

CASE CLOSED

4.7 Case 265 – "Marco"

Overview: Marco's case is a simple one, presenting with allergies and potentially with asthma. The DPT potency quickly did its job of eliminating a persistent cough, and higher potencies supported other treatment.

13.2.06 1st consultation

Marco was an 11-month-old boy who presented with allergies, especially to eggs. He gets hives if he touches an egg product. Both parents were allergic to shellfish. His mother is allergic to eggs.

Four weeks previously he started coughing. A doctor said it was a precursor to asthma.

He was vaccinated at 8 months of age.

He has only just started teething (none yet), but it hasn't been difficult so far. He walked early.

His sleep varies, with irregular waking. If he wakes regularly then he screams.

Generally, is a happy boy.

He has a strong personality. Seems laid back, but he can be very determined. If upset, he can throw himself on the ground and scream.

Appetite is very good, but doesn't put on weight. He is heat sensitive.

Rx. (1) DPT 10M fortnightly.

22.2.06 Sleep aggravated following remedy. Advised to wait.

3.4.06 (2nd consultation)
He has had two doses of (1). The coughing stopped.

He has developed a cold last Thursday, probably worse by teething.

His mother also said that he reacts very badly to mosquito bites.

Rx. (2) Calc Flour 200 every 2nd day as required to relieve teething.
To obtain the remedy Mosquito 30.

29.5.06 (3rd consultation)
Remedy (2) helped the teething a lot.
Marco has had 3 doses of (1) DPT 10M, which has stopped the coughing.

Rx. (3) DPT 50M, every 6 weeks.
(4) Calc Fluor M, to be used during teething.
(5) Mosquito 30, every 2 weeks when ready *(to desensitise him to mosquito bites – I have used this protocol very successfully in many sensitive patients).*

11.9.06 Marco is going very well, apart from the allergies to eggs.
Remedy (4) has helped greatly during teething.

Send (6) Ferrum Met 200, every 3 weeks *(this remedy has a similarity to egg allergies).*

CASE FINISHED

4.8 Treatment Failures

Nine cases were classified as T4 - patient worse. Table 19 summarises the major details of these cases. It is immediately clear that different potencies of the DPT vaccine were the remedies which aggravated. Skin problems were the most common problems which aggravated. In most cases the patients reacted to the potencies and stopped treatment. In others there was no immediate improvement, and parents moved on.

From a homoeopathic perspective, the fact that a remedy aggravates means that it also has the potential to assist. It also means that the patient was probably either given a potency which was too high, or was given too many doses, or simply that the patient had an abnormal sensitivity to any "similar" energetic stimulation. Of the six skin cases noted, four were started with a potency that was (with hindsight) too high. They were some of my earlier cases.

Only one of these nine patients came for a second consultation. This is also instructive for parents with vaccine injured children, as well as for adults who were injured as children. If a homoeopathic remedy causes an aggravation, then it also has the potential to fully deal with the cause of the problem, in this case vaccination. It is necessary at times to work with your practitioner, possibly for a year or more, to steadily reverse the vaccine injury.

Treatment is a partnership between the patient (and parents) and the practitioner. Treatment works best when there is cooperation and open communication.

Remedy aggravations also show clearly that homoeopathic potencies are not ineffective/inert placebos as suggested by many in orthodox medicine.

Table 19: Analysis of Treatment Failures

No	Main Initial Problem	Remedy	Result
66	Eczema	DPT M every 3 weeks	Eczema flared up, child not brought back.
67	Autism	DPT 200 fortnightly	Aggravated after the 2nd dose. Did not return.
175	Skin problems	DPT M single dose	No better after 1st dose. Took a 2nd dose and did not follow up.
226	Eczema	DPT M single dose	Skin worse after remedy. Did not follow up.
242	Spots on skin following reaction to vaccine.	DPT M weekly	Spots kept increasing. Stopped treatment.
244	ADHD – on Ritalin since grade 1	DPT M fortnightly	Got worse, is going back onto drug.
480	Skin at 3 months then regressed at 12 months	MMR 30, 200 Then DPT 30, 200, M, 10M	Cannot relax, constant noises, always on the go. Didn't worsen, but didn't improve.
539	Sensory issues, mild autism, worse change. Fearful.	MMR 200 Arsen 200	Had tried many other treatments. Was an email desperate case, and there was no immediate improvement. Will try other things.
753	Eczema from 6 mths	DPT 30, 200	Eczema worse after DPT200. No further follow-up.

Thirty-four other cases were classified as no improvement.

4.9 Final Cases

CASE D105: "Ruby"

This is a new case in the 4th edition, and I have selected it as an example of something that has become much more common since Covid – parents of children who don't appear to be unwell but who want their child to have a general vaccine detox.

Overview: Ruby's parents asked me to detox her. She appeared to be physically well, but did have temper tantrums at times, but these weren't clearly a consequence of vaccination. I started with the DPT detox, which had little effect, but when she began the MMR detox she had an immediate positive result. Not all reactions are negative, but all reactions indicate that the targeted vaccine is affecting the patient. The Infanrix HEXA remedies made little change, but as soon as MMR remedies started the improvement was immediate - meaning that Ruby was still affected by the MMR vaccine.

3/7/23
Ruby. - DOB: 04/05/2020 (3 years old)

Ruby had all vaccines from birth - 18 months. They were all on time, except the 18 month was given to her in Jan of 2022 instead of November 2021 (20 months old). Ruby's mother reported as follows:

"After 12 month vaccination (7 days after), she had what looked like mosquito bites on the back of her hand.
I believe it was the 18 month vaccination (can't be certain as I can't find a photo), she also had lots of tiny red bumps on the palm of her hand. I was told this was a reaction to body wash by doctors. It disappeared shortly after and never reappeared again.

- Formula fed as a baby, she had 'reflux' and used infant's friend with each bottle.
I had whooping cough taken during pregnancy

Physical:
- Looks to be a perfectly healthy 3 year old
- Having trouble staying asleep/Often waking in the middle of the night angry.

Emotional/mental:
- Easily agitated - Outbursts - Very reserved until she warms up to her environment (she does not attend daycare so this may contribute to this), which is not necessarily a bad thing.

Main reason for wanting a detox are her tantrums (think they started around 12 months of age). Can be intense. She is a very sensitive child.

Rx: (1) Hexa 200; (2) Hexa 50M; (3) MMR 200; (4) MMR 50M
To be given in order over 10 weeks unless reactions dictate a longer schedule. (1) and (3) twice a week for 2 weeks. (2) and (4) once a week for 3 weeks.

14/8/23 Ruby is currently on #3 of the vaccine detox. Her mother emailed:
"Changes I can see are:
- Immediately started sleeping better at night when starting the detox.
She does have the odd angry outburst when waking at night, however I feel that this happens after a day fuelled with sugar (after being at the grandparents etc). I see sleep improvements here.
- Outbursts during the day don't go for as long as usual. However, if they do, I can usually pinpoint the issue behind the behaviour (tired) etc.

Yesterday, she broke out in 3 pimples (not itchy) on her thighs (I have photos). That would be 2 days of tablets from #3 detox.
We did visit a farm the day before (unsure if related), touching animals? she was in cotton pants. So the fabric was not irritating."

27/8/23 Her mother emailed the following report: "Just a quick update for Ruby, she is currently on her first week of #4.
What I've noticed... Concentration levels, improved. I've noticed, she can play independently for longer periods of time.
Her creativity has just blossomed. She's less scared.
Less outbursts/not as often (when there is an outburst I can normally pinpoint why).
Sleep improved (we have popped her in her bed, and I sleep there with her little brother but I have noticed she's not waking angrily/not thrashing about at night)".

Ruby's case is not closed quite yet but should be soon. We may well use two more higher potencies of MMR to finish the case.

And my very last case in this 4th edition has occurred just as I was finishing off the final data collection for the book.

The case has only been going for a few weeks, and mostly cases take much longer to see results, but the email from John's mother came to me this morning, and it was such a positive and indeed joyful email I thought I would share it with you.

This is the reason why, despite having stopped taking on new general health cases, I am still taking on immunisation and vaccine injury cases. It is such a wonderful thing to see young lives turned around after being potentially damaged for life by vaccination.

CASE V895: "John"

21.8.2023. John was born on 18.6.2017.

He had all his standard vaccines up to 4 years of age. There were no immediate reactions, but he slowly stopped talking and development became delayed. He stopped speaking just before 2 years of age. He had poor eye contact from around 18 months of age.

NOW - he attends a special school which he loves because the teachers let him do his own thing. He prefers teachers to contact with other students. He will listen to simple instructions.

He loves music and nursery rhymes. Is in his own world, and often doesn't acknowledge others. But he is very affectionate with his own immediate family.

Loves playing with trains and leggo. Loves his iPad and is good with technology.

Rx: (1) MMRV 200, weekly dose. (2) MMRV 50M, dose to be advised (MMRV was chosen because that was the main vaccine at 18 months of age).

8.9.2023. Mother's email advised the following:

"Just wanted to update you about John's progress since starting his detox 2 weeks ago.

Today was his third week taking 2 tablets 1 x a week and we have noticed a dramatic difference. The difference my husband and I noticed was from the first week.

Here are what we have noticed:

He is more alert (he listens to our instructions and is making more eye contact)

Hasn't thrown any tantrums like he use to (he used to cry for no reason, but he hasn't done that since starting the detox)

Sleeps easily (he falls asleep more easily as he is more calm and quiet)

Doesn't overeat anymore (we were worried about his weight but now he is no longer looking overweight)

He is not toilet trained but his teacher told us he did his first poo in the toilet within the first week of starting his detox.

There are all positive and obvious signs we have noticed with John, and we cannot wait to see him improve even more."

And God Willing John will improve even more!!

5.1 General Conclusion

We set out to answer four questions, and I believe that they have been answered in the following way:

Q1. Do vaccines cause injury?
A. Yes. Not every time, and not in all people, but they do at times, and it is impossible to know in advance if they will and, if they do, how severe or long lasting that injury will be.

Q2. What are the symptoms of vaccine injury?
A. Many and varied, and on every level – mental, emotional, and physical. They include both short-term and long-term injury. They can range from death to slight swelling around the injection site, but the most common injury is a long-term destruction of the patient's general wellbeing; and a possible increase in a wide range of chronic conditions.

Q3. How can we prevent vaccine injury?
A. There is only one **certain** way – don't be vaccinated. Homoeopathic immunisation is available as a safe and comparably effective option.

Q4. How do we treat vaccine injury?
A. A patient suffering from vaccine injury can be assisted in many ways and by every modality. However homoeopathic medicine has a central role to play because it can both target the fundamental cause of many problems, and go back months, years, even decades to help eliminate residual injury caused by vaccination.

To my homoeopathic colleagues, I hope that the information presented here will assist you in recognising the symptomatic influence of different vaccines and give you information on treatment options available.

Personally, I can state without any hesitation that some of my most satisfying cases involved helping vaccine injured children regain their quality of life, and their suffering families their peace of mind.

5.2 A Personal Conclusion

I am often asked the following question: in the light of the results from all of this data concerning vaccination injury, and the potential value of homœoprophylaxis as an option to vaccination, then why doesn't the Government do something to support parents whose children have been injured, and support parents who want to use homoeopathic immunisation instead of vaccination?

This is a question you need to ask politicians.

I have tried at times in the past to communicate with State and Federal Health Ministers, but all my attempted communications were intercepted by their minders who were also people with orthodox medical training. The minders replied with nonsensical bureau-speak. The sad fact is that most politicians are intellectually captive to the pharmaceutical lobby, fronted as it is by distinguished Professors of Medicine, and medical researchers who dazzle the media and the politicians with their latest amazing discoveries.

You may have gathered from some of my comments that I find it hard at times not to be cynical and tremendously disappointed by the current state of affairs.

I live in one of the most blessed countries on the planet. We are blest with natural resources, general economic prosperity (which is not uniformly shared), a high level of tolerance (despite a fair sprinkling of racists and bigots), and most importantly with peace within our borders.

Yet we are chronically unhealthy as a nation. Despite being "sports-mad" we have recently passed the USA as the most obese country on earth (obviously more people are spectators than participants). As our health system moves closer to that of the USA, our levels of chronic illness across all age groups reach overwhelming proportions.

Our health system is almost completely controlled by multinational pharmaceutical interests, whose PR machine overwhelms voices of concern through a buy-out of the media in this country who have readily traded profits for integrity and independence. Any doubts about the truth of this statement were answered by the appalling Covid response from 2020 to 2023.

This media machine has convinced politicians of all parties to subsidize drugs and associated treatments to the tune of hundreds of millions of dollars each year. In America the cost runs into billions of dollars annually, which is not surprising because the pharmaceutical groups spend around 30 billion dollars annually in America in advertising, direct and indirect promotions, and on lobbying.

This control means that generations of otherwise well-intentioned medical practitioners have been taught to be totally closed minded to all except their own experience of the world. Unlike in much of Europe, many Australian doctors are against most forms of natural medicine simply because that is what they were taught in medical school.

This approach is of course totally unscientific. True science looks at all options objectively and without preconceptions.

All this means just one thing – until there appear some truly open-minded and courageous politicians who can think independently of their minders, it will be up to individual parents to make their own decisions about their own health and that of their children. There are a few encouraging signs that this is starting to happen, even if it is driven by the economic necessity of forging balanced budgets in later years as the population ages. Covid also opened many eyes for the first time.

Every book I have written has been to serve the purpose of informing parents – after all I am one myself, quite a few times over. This book is no different in intention. Some, including this book, have also been aimed at practitioners in all modalities, including those from orthodox medicine, to hopefully assist them to assist their patients.

I am still learning. I don't know it all, and never will. I have a great belief in the universal Law of Balance (some call it kharma and dharma - others simply call it justice). I believe absolutely that truth will always win in the end. I hope this modest offering will assist your search for the truth.

PART 4: Resources and Appendices

6.1 Useful Resources

Books

The following selected list of reference material relating to vaccination and children.

Books

Golden I. *Immunisation Options for Parents Who Care.* Isaac Golden Publications, Gisborne, Victoria. 2015.

Golden I. *The Complete Practitioners Manual of Homœoprophylaxis.* Isaac Golden Publications, Gisborne, Victoria. 2017.

Golden I, *Vaccination & Homœoprophylaxis? - A Review of Risks and Alternatives.* 7th ed. 2010. Isaac Golden Publications, Gisborne, Victoria. Revised 2007.

Golden I, *Homœoprophylaxis - A Practical and Philosophical Review.* 4th ed. Isaac Golden Publications, Gisborne, Victoria 2007.

Golden I, *Homœoprophylaxis – A Fifteen Year Clinical Study.* Isaac Golden Publications, Gisborne, Victoria. 2004.

Barham-Floreani J. *Well Adjusted Babies.* 2nd Edition. Vitality Productions Pty Ltd, Mt Macedon, Australia. 2009

Jordan L, *Challenging Children – Success With Homoeopathy.* Harbord Homoeopathic Childrens Clinic, Brookvale, NSW. 2007.

Australian Vaccination Network. *Vaccination Roulette: Experiences, risks and alternatives.* AVN, Bangalow, New South Wales. 1998.

Neustaedter R, The Vaccine *Guide: Risks and Benefits for Children and Adults.* North Atlantic Books. Berkeley, California. 2002.

Wilson G, *Vaccination and Behavioral Disorders.* Tuntable Creek Publishing. Lismore. New South Wales. 2000.

Coulter H L & Harris B, *D.P.T. - A Shot in the Dark*. Warner Books. New York. 1985.

Kalokerinos A, *Every Second Child*. Nelson. Melbourne. 1974.

Mendelsohn R S, *Confessions of a Medical Heretic.* Warner Books, Chicago. 1979.

Scheibner, V, *Vaccination: The Medical Assault on the Immune System.* 1993

Mendelsohn R S, *How to Raise a Healthy Child ... In Spite of Your Doctor*. Contemporary Books, Chicago, 1990.

Mothering Magazine. *Vaccinations. The Rest of the Story*. PO Box 1690, Sante Fe, NM 87504, USA.

Coulter H L, *Vaccination, Social Violence and Criminality. The Medical Assault on the American Brain.*

Websites

National Vaccine Information Centre (USA based, but excellent information). Founded by Barbara Loe Fisher. https://www.nvic.org/

Dr Smits website is a "must" for anyone interested in this topic. See: http://www.tinussmits.com/3734/home.aspx

The Australian Vaccination-Risks Network (AVN) has a website full of useful information. www.avn.org.au (This website is under attack at time of writing - but I managed to access via https://avn.org.au/information/vaccine-laws/)

Children Health Defense - led by Robert F Kennedy Jr. The new Australian Chapter is at https://childrenshealthdefense.org.au/

7.1 Appendices

Appendix 1: NVICP Compensation Data, 2019

Appendix 2: Vaccine Programs Worldwide

Appendix 3: Tinus Smits' Recommendations

Appendix 4: Australian Vaccination Support Groups

Appendix 5: International Vaccination Support Groups

Appendix 6: A Brief Explanation of Homoeopathy

Appendix 1: NVICP Compensation Data, 2019

NVICP	-	National Vaccine Injury Compensation Program
DHHR	-	US Department of Health and Human Resources
HRSA	-	Health Resources and Services Administration

Government official statistics, May 2019

http://www.hrsa.gov/vaccinecompensation/ (accessed 17/7/19).
https://www.hrsa.gov/sites/default/files/hrsa/vaccine-compensation/data/monthly-stats-may-2019.pdf (accessed 17/7/19).

Since 1988, over 20,629 petitions have been filed with the VICP. Over that 30-year time period, 17,875 petitions have been adjudicated, with 6,551 of those determined to be compensable, while 11,324 were dismissed. Total compensation paid over the life of the program is approximately $4.1 billion.

Petitions Filed, Compensated and Dismissed, by Alleged Vaccine, Since the Beginning of VICP, 10/01/1988 through 5/01/2019

Vaccines	Filed Injury	Filed Death	Filed Grand Total	Compen-sated	Dis-missed
DTaP-IPV	11	0	11	3	3
DT	69	9	78	26	52
DTP	3,286	696	3,982	1,273	2,709
DTP-HIB	20	8	28	7	21
DTaP	454	82	536	225	252
DTaP-Hep B-IPV	86	37	123	41	53
DTaP-HIB	11	1	12	7	4
DTaP-IPV-HIB	43	21	64	14	30
Td	206	3	209	123	75
Tdap	700	6	706	361	72

Tetanus	138	2	140	75	47
Hepatitis A (Hep A)	104	7	111	56	32
Hepatitis B (Hep B)	696	60	756	275	419
Hep A-Hep B	33	0	33	16	5
Hep B-HIB	8	0	8	5	3
HIB	44	3	47	18	20
HPV	393	15	408	130	167
Influenza	5,087	170	5,257	2,939	478
IPV	268	14	282	8	269
OPV	282	28	310	158	152
Measles	143	19	162	55	107
Meningococcal	79	2	81	44	8
MMR	980	61	1,041	402	584
MMR-Varicella	51	2	53	21	13
MR	15	0	15	6	9
Mumps	10	0	10	1	9
Pertussis	4	3	7	2	5
Pneumococcal Conjugate	194	16	210	53	50
Rotavirus	94	5	99	59	23
Rubella	190	4	194	71	123
Varicella	103	9	112	64	30
Nonqualified1	100	9	109	3	101
Unspecified2	5,426	9	5,435	9	5,399
Grand Total	**19,328**	**1,301**	**20,629**	**6,551**	**11,324**

Petitions Filed

Fiscal Year	Total		Fiscal Year	Total
FY 1988	24		FY 2004	1,214
FY 1989	148		FY 2005	735
FY 1990	1,492		FY 2006	325
FY 1991	2,718		FY 2007	410
FY 1992	189		FY 2008	417
FY 1993	140		FY 2009	397
FY 1994	107		FY 2010	448
FY 1995	180		FY 2011	386
FY 1996	84		FY 2012	401
FY 1997	104		FY 2013	504
FY 1998	120		FY 2014	633
FY 1999	411		FY 2015	803
FY 2000	164		FY 2016	1,120
FY 2001	215		FY 2017	1,243
FY 2002	958		FY 2018	1,238
FY 2003	2,592		FY 2019	709
			Total	**20,629**

Adjudications

Generally, petitions are not adjudicated in the same fiscal year as filed. On average, it takes 2 to 3 years to adjudicate a petition after it is filed.

Fiscal Year	Compen-sable	Dismissed	Total
FY 1989	9	12	21
FY 1990	100	33	133
FY 1991	141	447	588
FY 1992	166	487	653

FY 1993	125	588	713
FY 1994	162	446	608
FY 1995	160	575	735
FY 1996	162	408	570
FY 1997	189	198	387
FY 1998	144	181	325
FY 1999	98	139	237
FY 2000	125	104	229
FY 2001	86	88	174
FY 2002	104	104	208
FY 2003	56	100	156
FY 2004	62	247	309
FY 2005	60	229	289
FY 2006	69	193	262
FY 2007	82	136	218
FY 2008	147	151	298
FY 2009	134	257	391
FY 2010	180	329	509
FY 2011	266	1,740	2,006
FY 2012	265	2,533	2,798
FY 2013	369	649	1,018
FY 2014	370	192	562
FY 2015	517	137	654
FY 2016	697	179	876
FY 2017	696	185	881
FY 2018	540	189	729
FY 2019	270	68	338
Total	**6,551**	**11,324**	**17,875**

Awards Paid

Fiscal Year	No. of Comp-ensated Awards	Petitioners' Award Amount	Attorneys' Fees/Costs Payments	Total Outlays inc. Attorney paymt (dismissed cases)
FY 1989	6	$1,317,654.78	$54,107.14	$1,371,761.92
FY 1990	88	$53,252,510.46	$1,379,005.79	$54,689,215.73
FY 1991	114	$95,980,493.16	$2,364,758.91	$98,842,061.28
FY 1992	130	$94,538,071.30	$3,001,927.97	$98,752,676.41
FY 1993	162	$119,693,267.87	$3,262,453.06	$125,402,993.98
FY 1994	158	$98,151,900.08	$3,571,179.67	$104,889,607.13
FY 1995	169	$104,085,265.72	$3,652,770.57	$110,014,172.61
FY 1996	163	$100,425,325.22	$3,096,231.96	$105,885,679.89
FY 1997	179	$113,620,171.68	$3,898,284.77	$119,397,874.59
FY 1998	165	$127,546,009.19	$4,002,278.55	$133,484,353.24
FY 1999	96	$95,917,680.51	$2,799,910.85	$101,024,548.76
FY 2000	136	$125,945,195.64	$4,112,369.02	$131,782,015.74
FY 2001	97	$105,878,632.57	$3,373,865.88	$111,318,723.12
FY 2002	80	$59,799,604.39	$2,653,598.89	$63,109,448.07
FY 2003	65	$82,816,240.07	$3,147,755.12	$87,509,650.06
FY 2004	57	$61,933,764.20	$3,079,328.55	$66,211,708.71
FY 2005	64	$55,065,797.01	$2,694,664.03	$59,551,048.33
FY 2006	68	$48,746,162.74	$2,441,199.02	$52,540,994.37
FY 2007	82	$91,449,433.89	$4,034,154.37	$97,175,608.51
FY 2008	141	$75,716,552.06	$5,191,770.83	$83,556,982.40
FY 2009	131	$74,142,490.58	$5,404,711.98	$85,345,704.64
FY 2010	173	$179,387,341.30	$5,961,744.40	$189,261,439.67
FY 2011	251	$216,319,428.47	$9,572,042.87	$233,482,659.44
FY 2012	249	$163,491,998.82	$9,241,427.33	$186,803,360.70
FY 2013	375	$254,666,326.70	$13,543,099.70	$276,676,893.56
FY 2014	365	$202,084,196.12	$12,161,422.64	$223,563,646.17
FY 2015	508	$204,137,880.22	$14,445,776.29	$225,219,939.33
FY 2016	689	$230,140,251.20	$16,225,881.12	$252,610,672.33
FY 2017	706	$252,245,932.78	$22,045,785.00	$282,096,906.34
FY 2018	522	$199,658,492.49	$16,658,440.14	$226,628,298.86
FY 2019	358	$139,197,277.46	$10,014,749.86	$154,754,168.99
Total	**6,547**	**$3,827,351,438.68**	**$197,086,696.28**	**$4,142,954,814.88**

NOTE: Some previous fiscal year data has been updated as a result of the receipt and entry of data from documents issued by the Court and system updates which included petitioners' costs reimbursements in outlay totals, "Compensated" are petitions that have been paid as a result of a settlement between parties or a decision made by the U.S. Court of Federal Claims (Court). The # of awards is the number of petitioner awards paid, including the attorneys' fees/costs payments, if made during a fiscal year. However, petitioners' awards and attorneys' fees/costs are not necessarily paid in the same fiscal year as when the petitions/petitions are determined compensable. "Dismissed" includes the # of payments to attorneys and the total amount of payments for attorneys' fees/costs per fiscal year. The VICP will pay attorneys' fees/costs related to the petition, whether or not the petition/petition is awarded compensation by the Court, if certain minimal requirements are met. "Total Outlays" are the total amount of funds expended for compensation and attorneys' fees/costs from the Vaccine Injury Compensation Trust Fund by fiscal year. Since influenza vaccines (vaccines administered to large numbers of adults each year) were added to the VICP in 2005, many adult petitions related to that vaccine have been filed, thus changing the proportion of children to adults receiving compensation.

Pre-1988 Statistics Report - August 21, 2007

The Pre-1988 statistics report as of August 21, 2007 contains complete data on the number of claims filed, compensated, and dismissed as well as the number and amount of awards paid by fiscal year since the inception. Pre-1988 claims allege injuries from vaccines administered prior to October 1, 1988, the day the VICP began. Pre-1988 claims had to be filed by January 31, 1991.

I. Petitions Filed

Fiscal Year	Number Filed
FY 1988	24
FY 1989	147
FY 1990	3,199
FY 1991	864
FY 1992 - 2007	30
Total	**4,264**

II. Adjudications

Fiscal Year	Compensable	Dismissed	Totals
FY 1989	9	12	21
FY 1990	96	34	130
FY 1991	132	425	557
FY 1992	136	444	580
FY 1993	103	531	634
FY 1994	121	403	524
FY 1995	112	524	636

FY 1996	112	330	442
FY 1997	129	146	275
FY 1998	91	109	200
FY 1999	60	66	126
FY 2000	57	29	86
FY 2001	18	7	25
FY 2002	8	5	13
FY 2003	4	3	7
FY 2004	1	2	3
Totals:	**1,189**	**3,070**	**4,259**

III. Awards Paid (Petitioner's Awards AND Attorney's Fees Only Payments)

Fiscal Year	Number of Awards	Amount ($ in Millons)
FY 1990 - 1995	1,583	$496,104,984.48
FY 1996	278	$75,677,945.58
FY 1997	227	$72,528,592.59
FY 1998	183	$79,938,786.40
FY 1999	123	$51,350,425.66
FY 2000	96	$71,606,015.24
FY 2001	31	$36,084,950.38
FY 2002	10	$4,875,239.46
FY 2003	8	$12,485,292.69
FY 2004	3	$1,866,870.89
Totals:	**2,542**	**$902,519,103.37**

- The average pre-1988 injury award since inception is $849,237.

Claims Filed and Compensated or Dismissed by Vaccine[1]
February 4, 2008

Vaccines Listed in Claims as Reported by Petitioners

Vaccine(s)	Filed			Compensated	Dismissed
	Injury	Death	Total		
DT (diphtheria-tetanus)	61	9	70	19	47
DTP (diphtheria-tetanus-whole cell pertussis)	3,280	694	3,974	1,263	2,672
DTP-HIB	16	8	24	3	19
DTaP (diphtheria-tetanus-acellular pertussis)	227	58	285	69	93
DTaP-Hep B-IPV	16	7	23	2	3

DTaP-HIB	5	1	6	3	0
Td (tetanus-diphtheria)	115	1	116	49	51
Tdap	1	0	1	0	0
Tetanus	56	2	58	20	29
Hepatitis A (Hep A)	10	0	10	0	2
Hepatitis B (Hep B)	518	45	563	92	243
Hep A- Hep B	4	0	4	1	1
Hep B-HIB	3	0	3	1	1
HIB (*Haemophilus influenzae* type b)	15	3	18	6	5
HPV (human papillomarvirus)	0	0	0	0	0
Influenza (Trivalent)	187	14	201	20	20
IPV (Inactivated Polio)	259	14	273	6	264
OPV (Oral Polio)	279	26	305	157	146
Measles	142	19	161	54	107
Meningococcal	2	0	2	0	0
MMR (measles-mumps-rubella)	733	51	784	276	325
MMR-Varicella	5	0	5	0	0
MR	15	0	15	6	9
Mumps	10	0	10	1	9
Pertussis	5	3	8	2	6
Pneumococcal Conjugate	21	3	24	5	12
Rotavirus	30	1	31	20	11
Rubella	189	4	193	69	123
Varicella	38	2	40	18	12
Nonqualified[2]	58	7	65	0	64
Unspecified[3]	5,130	5	5,135	0	406
TOTAL	**11,430**	**977**	**12,407**	**2,162**	**4,681**

[1]The number of claims filed by vaccine as reported by petitioners in claims since the VICP began on October 1, 1988, which have been compensated or dismissed by the U.S. Court of Federal Claims (Court). Claims can be compensated by a settlement between parties or a decision by the Court.

[2] Claims filed for vaccines which are not covered under the VICP.

[3] Insufficient information submitted to make a determination.

Appendix 2: Vaccine Programs Worldwide

Vaccine Injury Compensation Programs Worldwide: Geoffrey Evans, M.D. 9.3.06

http://www.hrsa.gov/vaccinecompensation/accvmin03-09-06.htm

(page checked 17/7/19 and found to be deleted. It can be accessed at https://www.researchgate.net/publication/12740713_Vaccine_injury_compensation_programs_worldwide accessed 17/7/19).

Dr. Evans provided information on worldwide vaccine injury compensation programs. His research began by individually surveying existing vaccine injury compensation programs in preparation for a VICP-sponsored workshop held in 2000. Managers from over a dozen programs in Canada, Western Europe and Asia attended the 2-day workshop in Washington. Survey results were presented the following year at the European Vaccine Manufacturer's Association in Brighton, UK. More recently, Dr. Evans contacted each of the programs to update the 2000 survey information. This updated information was presented in November 2005 at the 3rd Congress of the Asociacion Espanola de Vacunologia in Madrid. One additional program, Finland, came to his attention while obtaining the new data. Today's presentation mirrors what was presented at the Madrid meeting.

There are many similarities and differences in the various programs. They came about because of important public policy questions. First, what do you do when there are victims of unpredictable reactions to properly manufactured and administered vaccines? Second, who is responsible for compensating people who experience vaccine injuries? Should they be compensated? If so, who should pay for it? Should it be the vaccine company who may have manufactured the product correctly, but unanticipated the adverse effects of product, or the government who is responsible for protecting public health, or other sources (private health insurance or excise tax on vaccines)?

In the U.S., medical injuries and malpractice claims were handled in the civil tort system where negligence needs to be proven. Either the product was inadequately made, or it was administered negligently, or the patient was not warned of the possible side effects. However, the problem arises when there is no fault on the part of the manufacturer or the administrator.

Historically, outside the U.S., adult victims were commonly covered in most industrial accident programs which did not contain coverage for disability compensation. Children, however, were not covered under these programs, and there was no compensation for severe disabilities, loss of future earnings, and permanent injury or death.

Dr. Evans provided information on 14 vaccine injury compensation programs in other countries which were detailed by category in a 2-page table handout. In 1953, the German Supreme Court ruled that people who were injured by compulsory vaccine (at that time it was smallpox vaccine) were entitled to compensation. In 1960, Germany and France were providing compensation for the vaccine injured. In the 1970s, the following countries established compensation programs due to DTP vaccine concerns: Japan, Switzerland, Denmark, New Zealand, Sweden, and United Kingdom. In the 1980s, Finland, Quebec, United States, and Taiwan started compensation programs, and in 1990, Italy and Norway formed programs.

The reasons for the enactment of compensation programs varied. Basically, programs were created because people believed that the government had a responsibility to compensate those who were injured by vaccines. Another reason these programs were created was that injuries caused by vaccines are unique and should be dealt with separately from other types of injuries (i.e., from industrial accident injuries). In the U.S., Japan, and the U.K., concerns over injuries from the DTP vaccines resulted in public pressure to create a compensation program. Other reasons included trying to avoid costly trials, and providing more consistency in liability law outcomes and compensation. In Italy and some other countries, the medical community pressured the government to create a compensation program.

All countries, except Sweden and Finland, were enacted through administration on the national level. Germany and Switzerland enacted their programs on the state level which is responsible for determining eligibility in compensation outcome decisions, and deciding which vaccines are recommended for use. Japan enacted their program on a state and local level. New Zealand has a compensation system that requires its citizens to participate and give up their rights to sue for injuries, whether from drugs, vaccines, or other products or services. Participation in this program is mandatory. Individuals in high-risk professions pay more to the "Accident Rehabilitation and Compensation Insurance Corporation," which is setup as a quasi-governmental private enterprise.

Sweden's compensation program called the "Pharmaceutical Insurance" started in 1978 by companies marketing pharmaceutical products. Compensation is not decided under their judicial system. Finland has a program similar to Sweden. Denmark switched to a private insurance system in 2004.

The eligibility criteria for the compensation programs vary from country to country. The criteria reflect the specific needs and vaccine recommendations found in these countries. Most countries specify the type of vaccines that are given, whether it is compulsory, recommended, or voluntary; the date of vaccination, injury, or filing of the claim; and the type and severity of the continued effects of the injury. Some specify the setting where the vaccine is given, such as public, clinic, doctor's office, type of employment of healthcare worker, and citizen requirements.

The vaccines covered in these programs are usually recommended for routine use. Few countries have compulsory immunization. Most of the compensation programs covered vaccines given to children or those who are required to get vaccines for certain occupations and travel. France provides coverage for specific vaccines required for healthcare workers and health profession students. In Italy, persons who received the typhoid vaccine for professional reasons, and who travelled outside the country became eligible for compensation due to the 1992 legislation enacted which covered contaminated blood products.

In the U.S., there are no Federal vaccination mandates. There are 50 different state laws and nearly all of the 14 vaccines covered under the VICP are mandated in these states.

Some of the countries have different filing deadlines and limit coverage to a certain time period. In the U.K., claims could at one point be filed for injuries dating back to 1948. In the U.S., a pertussis vaccine claim was filed with the VICP dating back to 1918. There were also cases filed from vaccines administered in the 1930s and 1940s. Japan and Norway have no time limits for filing, and Germany's deadlines are determined by their Cantons.

In terms of compensable injuries, most countries are not very specific other than the U.S. In Taiwan, they used the U.S. Vaccine Injury Table to compensate injuries until two years ago. Currently, they require that the injury have a certain level of severity and have lasting effects. Often the decision to compensate is based on temporal association as well as current knowledge of vaccine reactions.

In most countries, claims are usually filed with the administrative entity at the national level and eligibility for compensation is determined at the same level. Decisions about compensation are done through an administrative process using internal reviews with some outside consultants. Some countries employ more formal evaluations bodies consisting of health and legal professionals as prescribed by law to evaluate their claims. In Quebec, the process for reviewing a claim consists of each party choosing a physician who will support their causation theories, and then both of these physicians choose a third physician in order to obtain a majority vote.

Most programs do offer flexibility in making causation decisions. Other than that, Dr. Evans was not able to determine more precisely the criteria upon which these decisions are made. Usually, if there is a suggestion in the literature of some significance and there is a reasonable temporal association, causation will be determined in favor of the injured party. Many of the western European countries have very different healthcare systems than in the U.S. Many have universal health insurance that covers people from when they are born until they die.

All programs allow claimants the right to appeal decisions against compensation. Almost all provide four categories of basic compensation similar to the benefits listed under industrial accident programs. The U.K. is the exception and has a provision for tax free lump sum payment of 100,000 pounds to ease the present and future burdens of those suffering from vaccine injury and their families. The types of benefits covered by most programs include: (1) medical costs for laboratory testing, therapy, hospital care; (2) disability pensions that can be based on lost earnings and long-term care costs, or based on the severity of the injury; (3) lost earnings for adults to care for a disabled child; and (4) injurys for pain and suffering.

France is very specific about compensation for emotional distress and loss of consortium. Other programs provide additional benefits based on the severity of the injury and degree of inconvenience and discomfort. They all provide some type of death benefit, either for the family to pay funeral costs or for loss of income. Germany and Denmark apply provisions of their industrial injury pension laws to vaccine injury victims. Some countries also allow individuals to supplement payments obtained from other forms of social assistance, while others disallow such practices. Japan allows an individual to obtain both government and social assistance benefits and private insurance if available. In the U.S., individuals are compensated for un-reimbursed expenses.

The funding sources for vaccine injury compensation programs differ among countries. About half are funded from the national treasuries. Private insurance provides funding for programs in Sweden, Finland, and Denmark. Some programs are funded by vaccine manufacturers.

Most of these programs allow the filing of civil actions in addition to obtaining compensation. However, some programs preclude individuals from obtaining benefits from both systems or reduce the amount of benefits obtained through civil action by the amount of benefits received under governmental programs. Denmark, Germany, U.K., and Switzerland do not allow civil suits to be filed.

There is great variability in the number of claims filed. In the U.K. and Japan, public awareness was high and affected the number of claims filed. The data from Japan reflects an increase in claims due to more public awareness and the Urabe mumps vaccine causing cases of aseptic meningitis, which has led to a significant percentage in compensation. Other factors affected the number of claims filed including population size, numbers of vaccines administered, the types of injuries covered, and the willingness of the public to utilize government programs versus other options.

Dr. Evans concluded that vaccine injury compensation programs outside of the U.S. are working well, but there is not much awareness of their existence. All exist solely in industrialized countries. The Pan American Health Organization has expressed interest in creating compensation programs for developing countries. However, in order to have a compensation program, a country must be able to afford to buy vaccines.

Appendix 3: Dr Tinus Smits' Recommendations

TINUS SMITS POST VACCINE SYNDROME

http://www.tinussmits.com/3734/home.aspx (accessed 17/7/19). A number of sites are available describing Dr Smits work. The material below was taken from an earlier posting, but is relevant)

PVS is essentially diagnosed on the basis of carefully chosen questions directed to the patient or his parents. The practitioner should always consider seriously a diagnosis of *post-vaccination syndrome* whenever the complaints started at the time of, or in the period following, vaccination and a treatment according to the method in this booklet should be implemented as a first line of approach. This is to obviate an endless and ill-fated stream of examinations and therapies. Where positive results are achieved the suspected diagnosis of PVS is confirmed. Only as a second resort, if the patient does not benefit fully from the treatment implemented, should a follow-up diagnosis be made. Case 4 illustrates how wearisome this process can be.

Because of its high degree of reliability and efficacy, this method offers an excellent opportunity for establishing the cause of certain illnesses. One can trace step by step the vaccine, medicine or illness that has caused the complaint. This scheme also allows us to find the cause of the often discussed **'Jungle syndrome'**, a syndrome which has claimed so many young soldiers as victim and for which traditional medicine can offer neither an effective diagnostic procedure nor a satisfactory therapy. The case of Johan, a 19-year-old seaman, is a clear example of such a diagnostic and therapeutic procedure. See case 5.

Treatment is with potentised vaccine. Usually the best method for chronic PVS is to administer this remedy at four different potencies on four consecutive days; the first day 30C, the second day 200C, the third day 1M and the fourth day 10M. In each case about 10 globules (diameter 6.72) are introduced directly into the mouth without any fluid to be drunk. The granules dissolve completely within one minute. It is advisable not to eat or drink or brush the teeth for half an hour before or after this administration to allow the medicament to act without interference. If the symptoms are aggravated after one of the four potencies it is always necessary to wait until the reaction is over before continuing treatment. In such cases the same potency is then repeated. This procedure is continued as long as necessary for the patient's reaction to cease, normally after one or two repeat doses. The series is then completed. It is also possible to treat a severe reaction with a solution of the 30C. For this, ten globules are dissolved in half a glass of water which is administered, a sip or teaspoonful at a time, for one or two days. The most common reaction is fever, which does not require further treatment. If the child is vulnerable, as for example as a result of serious vaccine-related complications or if oversensitivity is anticipated, each potency can be administered weekly. Severe reactions can similarly be treated by weekly repeats of the same potency until no reaction is clearly discernible. If the disorder has not completely cleared up after three weeks, the whole series can be repeated. One to three series is usually sufficient.

In acute cases the treatment is largely similar, differing only in that the preference in acute cases is given to aqueous solutions of a 30C or 200C as described above. This solution is administered at the rate of a sip or a teaspoonful an hour for a number of days; three doses are usually sufficient. See case 6, Ragma.

Even where the post-vaccination syndrome is of several years' standing it can still be treated successfully, as is shown by case 7, where the patient had suffered for eleven years, and case 8; with a prehistory of 17 years. In both cases the complaints were effectively fully cured.

PREVENTION

Homoeopaths used to recommend, and sometimes still do, Thuja 30C before vaccination. Personally, I have had unfortunate experiences with this and have never been able to confirm its efficacy. Paediatrician Yvonne Pernet has recommended Thuja 30C to the parents of all the children she has vaccinated for several years. When she stepped over to the preventive use of potentised vaccines the difference in the results was indisputable. There were patently fewer side-effects to vaccination with this novel method. In fact, the *energetic level becomes safeguarded* so it can no longer be disturbed by the vaccine. It is as if the organism is warned of the approaching 'artificial' illnesses and can therefore better maintain its balance. It must be remembered that chronic complaints can only occur because the deeper levels of our energy have been disturbed.

The procedure is as follows: two days before vaccination, give the potentised vaccine (e.g. DKTP) at 200C, about 10 small granules (globules), and repeat after vaccination, on the same day. The granules are of lactose and are absorbed quickly in the mouth. If there is to be no further vaccination for the time being, it is a good idea to administer the potentised vaccine a month later in increasing potencies of **30C**, **200C**, **1M** and **10M** on four consecutive days in order to correct any possible disturbance to the deeper energy levels. If, as can never be completely excluded, complications still occur despite these preventive measures, it is recommended that a solution in water of the 200C be given for three days at the acute stage and to repeat the whole series several weeks later. See case 9, Lisette.

RECOMMENDATIONS

Besides the preventive measures using potentised vaccine in the 200C dilution as described above, other means of prevention can lessen the risks from vaccination. In the first place this means being alert to signals from the child following vaccination. All too frequently it is assumed that all will be well and a following vaccine is administered unadvisedly.

Dr. Jean Elminger declares in his book *La médecine retrouvée*[3] that:

1. **vaccination is carried out too early;** in the sense that the new-born baby is building up his own cellular (general) defence and will pay for a shift towards humoral defence with a weakening of its immune system as a whole. It is interesting to note in this context that cot deaths have practically been eradicated[1] in Japan, where the whooping-cough vaccine is not given before two years of age.
2. **too many vaccines are administered together;** Economic considerations have dictated for several years now that an increasing number of vaccinations be given at the same time, e.g. MMR-D(K)TP or DKTP-HIB. Six or seven different vaccines at one time brings added risks; after all, one would not naturally contract six or seven diseases at the same time.
   The original notion was to give the HIB separately from the DKTP as a combination of the two would overburden the child. In practice this created organizational difficulties so it was decided to give DKTP and HIB together. Three-month-old babies are therefore given 15 vaccinations in two months. The child's defence mechanism at this age is undeveloped and vulnerable. The defences passed from mother to child are slowly breaking down and the child has to develop its own defences. It is therefore not surprising that the child experiences difficulty in coping with the heavy stimulation of its specific defensive mechanism caused by the combined disease germs, foreign proteins, chemical pollutants and additives all being pumped into its body within a short period. Consequently all sorts of chronic complaints stemming from weakened general defences occur at

this time. This way the child is forced to concentrate on the specific defence against the administered diseases and is not given the chance to develop its own more general defence mechanism. The general defences can even be seriously broken down, as is shown by the cases described. The necessity for vaccinating so young and so frequently in a period of vulnerability has never been demonstrated. Generally speaking, two D(K)TP vaccinations and one booster six months later should be sufficient for the first four years of life. (see case 15).

3. **vaccination is carried out too frequently;** The necessity for such an early and so frequent vaccination in such a vulnerable period of life has never been proved. Two vaccinations and one booster six months later should be enough for the first four years. (see case 16).
4. **vaccines cultivated on animal proteins are used, which also contain chemical additives that can excite allergies;** The preparation of safer vaccines without animal proteins or chemical additives is no easy matter. One possibility would be the fully synthetic preparation of vaccines. The first fully synthetic vaccine (against malaria), originating in Bolivia, is already being used on a small scale.

SUMMING UP I should like to make the following recommendations concerning vaccination policy.

1. **To implement vaccination later.** Hold back vaccination until the child has built up its cellular defences (general defences) sufficiently.
   There are enough variations worldwide in the age at which children receive their first vaccination for a preliminary balance-sheet of the advantages and disadvantages to be made up. A useful example is the whooping-cough vaccination in Japan, which is not given before two years[1]. A comparative study could be made by for example not vaccinating children from a particular region before ten months and following their progress compared with a control group of children vaccinated from their third month.
2. **To administer vaccines separately where possible.** In the first place the HIB can be given by itself again, as in the USA. Moreover the DKTP or DTP should never be combined with the MMR, as now happens with nine-year-olds. Vulnerable children who displayed strong reactions to an earlier vaccination should as a matter of course be given a DTP instead of a DKTP. Research[6] shows that DKTP gives more cause for complaint than DTP.
3. **Increase the intervals between vaccines:** two months instead of one month. This is less troublesome to the child and is more efficacious.

4. **Reducing the total number of vaccinations to three** from four for the D(K)TP and HIB, the first two with an interval of two months and the third after six months, as is already the case for children of foreign origin.
5. **Keeping a careful record of the child's reactions to the previous vaccine** before further vaccinating the child. A more stringent and cautious policy than the present one towards complications needs implementing.
6. **No further vaccinations before complete recovery** from post-vaccination symptoms. Children with a suspected post-vaccination syndrome require treatment and cure with the potentised vaccine. Following this, full or partial vaccination should be abandoned and preventive measures with the vaccine at 200K need to be taken.
7. **Systematic protection with potentised vaccine** at every vaccination if the comparative study yields positive results.
8. **Specific instruction** concerning PVS to doctors, nurses and parents.

Appendix 4: Vaccination Support Groups

A number of support groups exist in most countries, whereby experiences and concerns relating to vaccination may be shared. Some national groups do exist, and some are listed below. For anyone wanting an excellent summary of available links, I recommend the following Australian Vaccination Network (AVN) site - https://avn.org.au/information/useful-links/ (accessed 17/9/19)

Australia

Australian Vaccination-risks Network (AVN) - www.avn.org.au
PO Box 177 Bangalow NSW 2479. Ph. (02) 66871699

Vaccine Information Serving Australia Inc (VISA) -
www.visainfo.org.au (or https://www.facebook.com/VisaVaccinationInformationServingAustralia if website not available).
Vaccination Information South Australia formed on the 11th of February 1997, out of a need to respond to the government push to raise immunisation levels, and a need to provide alternative factual information about vaccination, including the dangers. We are a voluntary, non-profit, membership funded organisation. PO Box 643 Magill SA 5072. Ph. (08) 8336 5236. Email: visa@adelaide.on.net

Vaccination Awareness and Information Service (VAIS)
V.A.I.S. is a non-profit, volunteer organization dedicated to supplying factual information on vaccinations so parents can make an informed choice on this issue. We have a comprehensive health library and support groups in many areas so like-minded, health conscious parents can get together and support each other. Call Stephanie on 07 3821-5454 or 0412671922 for information or a support group near you. http://www.vaccinationawareness.com.au/ (accessed 17/7/19).
Email: growingawareness@hotmail.com

Vaccination Information Service - www.vaccination.inoz.com
For comprehensive information sourced from extensive literature including over 100,000 pages of medical research articles on vaccination collected by internationally recognised expert Dr Viera Scheibner, who has published a number of scientific papers in reputable scientific and medical journals. Also supportive information on legal rights and how to build strong immunity. Books, videos, DVD, colour information brochures and packs available.
PO Box 4. Turramurra. NSW 2074. Ph. (02) 9144 6625. Email: vaccinfo@bigpond.com

Healthy Families of Illawarra, Wollongong, Ph. (02)4284-6143. Kiama (02) 4232 1761

Australian Association for Humane Research Inc, PO Box 779, Darlinghurst NSW 2010

Campaign Against Fraudulent Medical Research, PO Box 128, Cabramatta NSW 2166

Appendix 5: International Vaccination Support Groups

New Zealand

Immunization Awareness Society (IAS) - http://www.ias.org.nz/

United States

National Vaccination Information Centre (NVIC) - https://www.nvic.org/ (accessed 17/7/19).
One of the best sites providing vaccine information. Barbara Lou Fisher is an outstanding person who speaks plainly and without embellishment about facts.
512 W. Maple Ave, Suite 206, Vienna, Virginia 22180, United States. Phone (703) 938-0342

Vaccine Information and Awareness (VIA) -
http://www.access1.net/via
792 Pineview Drive, San Jose, CA 95117, USA. (408) 448-6658

United Kingdom

Vaccine Information Service (VIS) - http://www.vaccine-info.com/ (accessed 17/7/19).

Special Mention

Finally, I would like to direct interested readers to an outstanding publication by Professor Brian Martin, ***Vaccination Panic in Australia***. Prof Martin is an academic of immense integrity and courage, as well as scholastic strength. His review of the situation regarding those who question vaccination in Australia is compelling reading. It is available online at a number of sites, including https://www.academia.edu/36388717/Vaccination_panic_in_Australia (accessed 17/7/19).

He supervised the Doctoral thesis of Dr Judy Wilyman. See https://vaccinationdecisions.net/about-us/ and https://ro.uow.edu.au/theses/4541/ (both accessed 17/7/19), which is also compelling reading.

NOTE: Some will say that my referencing of these resources proves I am an "anti-vaxxer". It doesn't, but that will not stop them making the claim. My purpose is to ensure that parents making decisions about infectious-disease-prevention have all sides of the discussion available to them, and the information supporting the pharmaceutical option is widely available. It is really difficult to find simple, unbiased information. This makes parental choice difficult for those caring parents who want to make an informed decision, rather than simply follow the unthinking majority.

I have the greatest respect for all parents who choose to think rather than blindly follow - whatever their final decision is.

I support many parents who contact me and who, for a variety of reasons, choose to vaccinate their children. All any caring parent can do is to collect relevant information and make the best decision they can for their child. Once you do that then proudly own that decision, because you have shown more love and care and concern than most.

Don't be intimidated by the mindless noise made by the ill-informed, or by those with vested interests, on any side of the debate. Not an easy task, but one which will prove the most important for your child's future.

Appendix 6: A Brief Introduction to Homoeopathic Medicine

1 - What is Homoeopathy?

Homoeopathy is a system of healing that was founded by a German physician, Dr Samuel Hahnemann. He actively began his work on his new system in 1790, and continued to his death in 1843, aged 88.

Hahnemann coined the term homoeo-pathy from two Greek words meaning *similar* (homois) *suffering* (pathos). He used "similar suffering" because homoeopathy is based on a Law of Nature which Hahnemann called the *Law of Similars*.

Hahnemann acknowledged that the Law was known to ancient healers such as Hippocrates. But he became the first to develop an accessible healing system that used the Law as its foundation.

Hahnemann knew of the *Law of Similars* through his medical studies but experienced it firsthand in 1790. At that time, he had almost given up the practice of medicine, and was making a living by translating medical texts into one of the seven languages in which he was fluent.

He was translating Cullen's *Materia Medica* (a book of mainly herbal remedies) from English into German when he disagreed with Cullen's description of the action of cinchona bark.

Hahnemann decided to take some of the bark twice daily for some days until he developed symptoms. In fact, the bark produced symptoms of fever with chilliness, thirst, flushing of the face and sleepiness. The symptoms ceased when he stopped taking the bark, but returned when he again took the bark.

Hahnemann knew that the symptoms he had developed were similar to symptoms of malaria. He also knew that cinchona bark was the source of quinine which is used to treat malaria.

Hahnemann realised that he had experienced the *Law of Similars* in practice – i.e. a substance that is capable of producing symptoms in a healthy person, is capable of removing similar symptoms in an unwell person.

The *Law of Similars* became the foundation of homoeopathic medicine.

Hahnemann then began conducting trials of different substances together with a few dedicated colleagues. These trials were called *provings*. Through these provings Hahnemann developed a unique collection of mental, emotional and physical symptoms for each substance, which became homoeopathy's own *Materia Medica*.

One reason why Hahnemann had stopped practicing medicine was because he was unhappy with the damaging toxic effects of the medicines commonly used. So when he began his new therapeutic system he also began experimenting to find the lowest possible dose of each remedy needed to produce a therapeutic effect.

He began diluting doses. Initially he found that the toxic side effects reduced without a loss of therapeutic benefit. But as the amount of dilution increased, a point was inevitably reached where the remedy stopped working.

Then Hahnemann did something which to this day has attracted praise from some, rebuke from others, as well as a continual question of "how did he know what to do?"

At each stage of dilution, Hahnemann began violently shaking the remedy container against a firm surface. He called this process *potentisation*. He found that not only did the toxic side effects of the initial substance disappear, but that the therapeutic action began to extend into the mental and emotional aspects of each case.

Potentisation has been condemned by many in pharmaceutical medicine as unscientific nonsense. The present orthodox paradigm cannot cope with concepts involving "energy" rather than physical substance. Fortunately, this is changing, and eventually quantum physicists may produce an explanation which satisfies a growing awareness of the full spectrum of life.

Potentisation will be explained in detail in Section 4 below.

Hahnemann then began using his new potencies, giving each patient only as much as they needed to produce a therapeutic effect. This method of dosing is based on another Law of Nature – the *Law of Minimum Dose*.

So, homoeopathy may be defined as a system of healing which selects remedies using the Law of Similars, and administers remedies using the law of Minimum Dose.

In the 1800's Hahnemann devoted the rest of his life to proving new remedies, experimenting with methods of preparing remedies, as well as investigating the true nature of disease.

In 1810 Hahnemann published the first of six editions of his *Organon of Medicine*, which provided both the philosophical basis of homoeopathy, as well as a practical "how to" set of rules for new homoeopaths to use.

In 1821 he published his *Materia Medica Pura* which described the symptoms of 62 proven remedies.

In 1828 Hahnemann published *Chronic Diseases*. This book was the result of 12 years of concentrated work to find the true cause of chronic disease. In it, Hahnemann developed his concept of *miasms*, which we shall examine later in the book.

Hahnemann was a truly amazing man. He built on a known, but little used, Law of Nature to produce a method that could assist in the healing of all levels – mental, emotional and physical – in a structured way, and without toxic side-effects.

He had to fight many bitter battles against dogma and entrenched self interests, to move the practice of medicine forward into a rational healing art and science.

His new ideas and developments were simply groundbreaking. Some of them are discussed in the following Chapter.

It is to the continual discredit of the orthodox medicine hierarchy, that medical students are not taught a complete and unbiased history of medicine. Our health system would be so much the better for it if they were.

2 - The Advantages of Homoeopathy

All the traditional ingestive modalities of natural medicine – herbs, tissue salts, flower essences, nutritional medicine, as well as homoeopathy, have much to offer.

Homoeopathic medicine has some special characteristics which differentiate it from the other modalities. The main differences are:

1. The Law of Similars

Homoeopathy is the only healing modality that intentionally and systematically uses the *Law of Similars* as the foundation of its method. Other therapies occasionally use the *Law of Similars*, either deliberately or unintentionally (for example, pharmaceutical medicine uses Ritalin (amphetamines or "speed"), to slow down hyperactive children). The great advantage of basing the entire healing system on an unchanging Law is that the implementation of the method remains the same over time. This is unlike pharmaceutical medicine, where treatments are based on a continually changing series of experiments, driven often by corporate profits.

2. Individualisation

More than most other healing modalities, homoeopathy requires a very high level of individualisation in order to select the most appropriate remedy. There are over 3,000 remedies in the homoeopathic *Materia Medica*, allowing for precise remedy-patient matching. There is a down-side to this need for individualisation – if the remedy selection is not accurate, the remedy will not work.

3. Provings

This unique method of testing and quantifying the healing potential of a substance can reveal all aspects (mental, emotional and physical) of the remedy, and it provides immensely valuable data for the practitioner. Without provings, the systematic use of the *Law of Similars* would not be possible.

4. Potentisation

Once again, this unique method of preparing medicines allows for treatment on all levels. It also enables a significant retracing of symptoms. For example, if a 50-year-old patient was traumatised when 5 years old, this old wound can be treated using highly potentised medicines.

5. Constitutions
Homoeopathy recognises that there are certain personality characteristics which appear to be unchanging over life. These characteristics form what is called the *constitution* of the patient, and can assist in finding a remedy that eventually will assist the patient to improve every aspect of their life.

6. Miasms
Hahnemann's ground-breaking research into the true cause of chronic disease allows the trained practitioner to understand many of the reasons **why** a patient is suffering their health problems, and then do something about it by using special remedies which can remove these chronic impediments to health.

As you can see, there are many positive aspects of homoeopathic medicine. This is not in any way suggesting that there is something wrong with other natural healing modalities – they all have wonderful and positive aspects which can contribute greatly to our quality of life.

But in homoeopathy you have a modality which is safe, effective on all levels, and inexpensive. A great blessing.

3 - The Real Meaning of Health and Disease

The main conceptual difference between natural medicine and pharmaceutical medicine rests with opposing concepts of health and disease.

Pharmaceutical medicine is essentially designed to remove the symptoms of defined diseases. It is not based on unchanging natural Laws, but upon ever changing models of how the body works. The disease and its symptoms are seen as being the problem, and the body is chemically or surgically influenced to remove the symptoms.

Natural medicine in general, and homoeopathy in particular, sees symptoms as signs of a deeper disorder. Medicines are given to assist the natural self-healing force to do the healing. Artificial suppression of symptoms is seen as something which can worsen the true inner disease.

Hahnemann had a challenging experience early in his homoeopathic career. He began working with the *Law of Similars* and found it was very successful; however, he then found that many patients, who had apparently been cured, returned in 6-12 months time with similar complaints.

Hahnemann realised that there must be a deeper disturbance or cause that the similar remedies were not treating. He then spent 12 years of his life researching the history of disease. Because he was fluent in seven languages, this meant studying records in Latin, Greek, Hebrew, Aramaic, English, French and German.

At then end of this time, Hahnemann produced his great work *Chronic Diseases*, in which he introduced the concept of *Miasms*. He saw Miasms as the true cause of chronic diseases. They were energetic disturbances which prevented the body's self healing power, the *Vital Force*, from doing what it always will do if allowed to act freely – to rebalance disturbances on the physical, mental and emotional levels.

So, homoeopaths see the patient's disease symptoms as being the **results** of the *Vital Force* trying to expel the true **causes** of ill health, the *Miasms*.

If we define "disease" in orthodox terms - i.e. a collection of symptoms/pathology called asthma, or diabetes, or nephritis, etc, then **disease is the result of the patient being deeply unwell**, rather than saying that the patient is unwell because of the disease.

To summarise:
1. We all have a God-given self-healing energy which homoeopaths call the *Vital Force*. If allowed to act freely, it will always return the patient to balance on the mental, emotional and physical levels when they become unbalanced by external stressors.
2. The *Vital Force* is prevented from acting freely by chronic disturbances called *Miasms*, which most homoeopaths see as being the true cause of chronic disease. Disease symptoms are actually the results of the *Vital Force* attempting to remove the *Miasms*, they are not causes.
3. The purpose of homoeopathic remedies is to remove the *Miasms* which are blocking the free action of the *Vital Force*. If successful, the *Vital Force* then returns the patient to balance on all levels.
4. It is always the patient's own *Vital Force* which produces the healing, not the remedy. The purpose of the remedy is to remove those things which impede the free action of the *Vital Force* (i.e. to remove the *Miasms* and related disturbances).

4 - Provings, Potentisation, and Remedy Administration

We shall now consider in more detail, remedy testing, remedy preparation, and remedy administration.

Provings

Provings are carefully controlled clinical trials made to uncover the symptoms that substances can cause in healthy people. Provings are essential to provide the remedy symptoms which must be matched with the patient's symptoms, as required by the *Law of Similars*.

These carefully run trials recruit healthy volunteers. If a person is too unwell, their illness may mask the action of the remedy.

The trial is overseen by a *Master Prover*. If conducted properly, the trial is "double blind" (neither the provers nor the master prover know what substance is being trialled) and "placebo controlled" (a medicinally neutral substance is given to some of the provers to provide a control group against which the symptoms produced by those proving the active substance can be measured).

Each prover is asked to begin a diary a week or two before commencing the proving, listing things such as their diet, and any health problems that they regularly experience. The latter must be removed from the eventual list of remedy symptoms, unless the remedy being proved actually heals the symptoms, which occasionally happens.

The selected substance, often in 30c potency, is taken. There are different ways to proceed here, but often a single dose is given. If symptoms appear, they are recorded over the following month. If not, then daily doses of the remedy are given until symptoms appear. Sometimes a prover will not produce symptoms, and the remedy is eventually stopped. The central rule of all provings is; once symptoms begin to appear, stop the remedy. If this direction is followed, then the proving will be safe.

Provers are directed to record all the symptoms that are produced in their diaries, showing not only the actual symptom in complete detail, but when it occurred, and what factors seemed to make the symptoms better or worse. If any other symptoms changed at the same time, they are also to be recorded.

After about a month the proving is stopped, and the master prover collects all the diaries from the provers. He or she then extracts the information and lists (i) new symptoms that most provers experienced, (ii) new symptoms which a few provers experienced, and (iii) new symptoms which only one or two provers experienced. This information provides the basis for the grading of symptoms that appear in our *Repertories*.

Provers are advised not to discuss any of their experiences during the proving with other provers. The amazing fact is that a group of strangers from around the world can take an unknown (to them) substance, and produce a similar group of symptoms. This demonstrates the strength and consistency of natural Law.

Potentisation

Hahnemann initially developed this unique method of remedy preparation to reduce the toxic side effects of medicinal substances. He then found that the more energetically active the substance became, the more deeply it would work in a patient – touching deep psychological traumas that occurred many years earlier, but which were still affecting the patient's health on all levels.

Let us use, as an example, the preparation of the remedy Pulsatilla.

One drop of plant juice is mixed with 99 drops of alcohol and water, and *successed* – firmly struck against a firm surface a number of times (10 to 30 times is common). This produces the first centesimal potency, or **1c**.

One drop of the **1c** potency is then mixed with 99 drops of alcohol and water, and successed again, making the second centesimal potency, or **2c**.

The process is repeated as often as required. The most common potencies used by Australian homoeopaths are **6c, 30c, 200c** and **1000c** (or **M**).

For solid or insoluble substances, Hahnemann used a method called *trituration*, which involved grinding the substance with milk sugar using a pestle and mortar. One part of substance was mixed with 99 parts of milk sugar, and triturated, making **1c**. And so on to **3c**, at which point the substance will be soluble, allowing potentisation of the substance in liquid form to the higher potencies.

When remedies are prepared in a homoeopathic laboratory, medicinal alcohol and triple distilled water is used. Cleaned and sterilised containers are used at every stage, and measurements are precise.

However, if you decide to make a potency of say Chamomile tea at home to treat teething symptoms, you can use alcohol purchased from a chemist, mixed with pure spring water, and use approximate measurements. An effective potency will still be produced.

Remedy Storage and Administration

Because homoeopathic medicines are prepared to utilise the energy of substances, they can be antidoted if not treated with care.

Remedies should be stored away from strong heat and light. They should be kept away from strong electrical fields such as power boxes, microwaves, TV's, as well as mobile phones. The bottle should never be opened in the presence of strong odours such as perfumes, liniment, essential oils, etc.

If pilules are used, it is best to tip 1 or 2 pilules onto the lid of the container, and from there into the mouth, where they should be allowed to dissolve. If the remedy is in liquid form, 5 drops can be placed directly into the mouth, and held for 30 seconds. Alternatively, the drops can be placed in half a glass of water, stirred vigorously, and then a teaspoon of liquid placed in the mouth and held for 30 seconds. Pilules may also be dissolved in water if preferred.

5 - Taking a Homoeopathic Case

The purpose of homoeopathic case taking is to discover the characteristic or unique symptoms of each patient.

Hahnemann gave very clear instructions in his *Organon of Medicine* as to how to take a homoeopathic case. If you become seriously interested in homoeopathy, then it is an inexpensive little book. It is not an easy read, as Hahnemann's writing style was demanding. However, his directions regarding case taking can be readily understood, and are worth studying many times.

I will begin with a brief summary of the way to take a homoeopathic case, and then will list Hahnemann's main rules. The numbers in brackets refer to the *aphorism* or paragraph in the *Organon*.

Basic Homoeopathic Case Taking

The purpose of case taking is not just to try to write down every possible symptom the patient has, but to find those symptoms that are most characteristic, peculiar and rare (*PQRS* symptoms as they are called). These are the symptoms of the patient, not just the disease.

The cases you will be treating will mainly be acute problems such as colds, fevers, influenza, stomach upsets, constipation and diarrhoea, and so on. However, *PQRS* symptoms will appear even in these relatively simple cases. They are often the key to finding the most similar remedy.

Hahnemann first advised us to allow patients to tell us their story with a minimum of interruption, so as not to break their train of thought, and thus loose valuable symptoms that otherwise would emerge.

We should use plenty of paper. Write down a symptom, and leave space below it so that we can come back later and ask more questions to find its location, sensations, modalities and concomitants.

Always try to find out **why** a symptom is there. Recording **when** each symptom first appeared will give us valuable information to help us find the why. For example, we might find that a rash which troubles the patient began in May of 2002. We may later learn that the patient's daughter left home in March 2002 to attend College. This might suggest that the rash really was caused by the patient's concern for their daughter's welfare, and by the separation. This will lead to a completely different remedy being chosen than if the rash was caused by say brushing against stinging nettle, even though the symptoms of the rash may be similar. This is what we mean by – *treat the patient, not the disease*.

Any external causes, or *maintaining causes* as Hahnemann called them, need to be identified. If a patient's mucus problems are worsened by damp and mould, and they live in a damp, mouldy house, then the needed remedy may be to leave the house. If that is not possible, then the remedies may only be able to offer superficial relief whilst the patient is constantly exposed to the aggravating factor.

Try to ask questions that will encourage the patient to answer in their own language, rather than by "yes" or "no". For example, don't ask "do you dislike really cold weather?" Most people will say "yes", but this doesn't help us a lot. Instead ask "what type of weather do you dislike?" This makes the patient tell their own story in their own words. They might say "I don't particularly like the cold, but I am OK if I rug up. I enjoy warm weather, but if it gets too hot I get headaches, and feel really tired". This gives us useful information about the patient.

Case taking is a science and an art. The more you do, the better you will become, provided of course that you can objectively analyse your own performance. You often learn a lot about yourself as well as the patient during a well taken case. Even for the simple conditions you will be analysing, you will never stop learning to improve your case taking.

Remember always - **find the why**!

Hahnemann's directions for case taking are in the 6th edition of the *Organon of Medicine*, and are shown in Aphorisms (paragraphs) 84 to 104 for those readers who would like to know more.

6 - Analysing the Information from the Patient

Once the case has been carefully taken, the information must be analysed in order to uncover the best remedy. There are essentially six methods of homoeopathic prescribing with their associated methods of analysis. The first three focus mainly on symptoms, while the second three focus mainly on the patient as a unique individual. More detail about this second approach (prescribing for the patient) will be discussed in Chapter 7. The six methods are shown below:

Method 1: Use of a disease-specific complex remedy. The analysis here is quite superficial. The "name" of the disease is noted, the remedy for the disease is looked up in a product manual, and the remedy given.

For example, if a patient presents with asthma, the prescriber looks up "asthma" in the product manual and prescribes the remedy listed under that disease. It is usually a remedy which contains a number of related homoeopathic medicines mixed together, and patented under a specific product name (such as "asthmaplex", or something similar).

Homoeopaths of course believe that such prescribing is not true homoeopathy. The individualising symptoms of the case are not considered, no attempt is made to find the most similar remedy, and the symptom profile of the combination remedy (usually referred to as a *complex*) is rarely ever proved. This method is seen as being a "shotgun" approach – i.e. if enough bullets (remedies) are fired, one is sure to have some effect.

At times, the combination remedy brings symptomatic relief to the patient. Some homoeopaths believe that this relief is only superficial, and the remedy is almost certainly not going to heal the disease.

Method 2: Analysis using a *Prescriber* to select a disease-specific single remedy. In this method a single remedy is used, rather than a combination remedy. The remedy is selected by choosing between a number of single remedies, all of which are known to be indicated in many cases of the condition affecting the patient. This method does utilise the *Law of Similars* by using proved remedies. The method works reasonably well in simple conditions provided that Method 3 (below) is used IF the remedies listed in the *Prescriber* don't fit the patient's symptoms well.

Method 3: Analysis of mainly physical symptoms using repertorial analysis. In this approach we are concentrating on the physical complaints of the patient. We are now using a more sophisticated method of choosing the most similar remedy, which involves the following:

1. The patient's main symptoms are listed.
2. They are looked for in a book of symptoms called a *Repertory*. If the symptom is present, it is listed in a matrix or grid (in the *Repertory*, the symptom is called a *rubric*). The matrix shows how many rubrics each remedy covers, and the weight (or relative importance) of the remedy as it relates to each symptom.
3. From the repertorial matrix, a short-list of remedies that appear to have a degree of similarity to the patient's symptoms is prepared.
4. The short-listed remedies are examined in the *Materia Medica*, and the most similar is chosen. The potency and frequency of administration is then decided.

This approach clearly relies on the *Law of Similars*, however it generally limits the analysis to the main physical symptom(s) of the patient.

Method 4: Complete analysis of mental, emotional and physical symptoms using repertorial analysis. This method uses the same analytical structure as Method 3, except that in this case not only the physical symptoms are considered, but the mental/emotional, or personality symptoms of the patient as well.

As before, the *Repertory* provides a guide into the *Materia Medica*, which is where the final decision is made, based on the comparison of all of the patient's symptoms with all of the symptoms of the short-listed remedies.

Method 5: Constitutional analysis. In this method we are looking past the simple listing of individual symptoms to an *essence* that can be perceived in the totality of symptoms. We call this essence of the patient their *constitution*. This represents the personality profile of the patient – their characteristics as a unique individual. In depth knowledge of many remedies and remedy groups is needed to make an accurate constitutional prescription.

Method 6: Miasmic analysis. This method requires the homoeopath to once again see behind the simple listing of individual symptoms, and to perceive the presence of the miasmic disease entity, which Hahnemann saw as the true cause of chronic disease. It takes many years of study and experience to fully understand how to recognise the miasms, and how to treat them appropriately.

The purpose of all these analyses is to find the most similar remedy – the *similimum*.

When you first begin prescribing, you will mainly use method 2 – the *Prescriber* which comprises Part 1 of this series, or a similar book.

If you find that you really enjoy the experience and want to do more and better, then you will need to learn how to use a *Repertory* and a *Materia Medica*. Part 2 of this series gives a very simple example of both, but it is a start only. The *Intermediate Course* offered by the Australasian College of Hahnemannian Homoeopathy is a suitable next step to perfect your basic skills, including how to construct a repertorial matrix to use in case analysis.

To use the more sophisticated methods (4-6) requires professional training.

7 - Treating the Patient, Not the Disease

There is an old saying in homoeopathic circles – "treat the patient, not the disease". We have mentioned this a few times already.

Behind this saying is the understanding that the true cause of most diseases occurs on a more subtle level than the physical level on which many symptoms appear.

For example, a child may develop asthma following an emotional trauma. An adult may suffer from insecurity and depression as a result of being unloved by one or both parents. Another may suffer from fatigue and recurring glandular infections ever since a bad disease.

These are simple examples of what we call *never well since* events – a patient whose health has never been the same since a physical, emotional, or mental trauma. This relates to the aetiological similimum mentioned in Chapter 8 following.

If we only treat the obvious presenting symptoms, we may give temporary relief to the patient but the problems may keep recurring. Until we treat the cause, the results will continue. Until we treat the whole person, the parts of the person may continue to be disturbed.

When you begin homoeopathic prescribing, most of your cases will be simple physically-based problems – coughs, colds, constipation, minor wounds, travel sickness, and so on.

However, it is always possible to look behind the obvious and search for deeper causes. One of the most effective ways of doing this is to carefully note down **when** problems began. **Timing is everything** in uncovering the real causes.

For example, a 40-year-old adult may have suffered from annoying rashes for 15 years. A careful analysis of the rash may suggest the remedies *Sulphur, Psorinum* and *Natrum Muriaticum. Sulphur* is clearly the most similar, and therefore is prescribed first. The remedy helps a little but is clearly not the needed remedy.

With such an incomplete result, it is then appropriate to take the case again. You might find that the patient had a rash from 12 months of age to 5 years old. He then was healthy for many years. He married when he was 20 but lost his wife in a tragic accident when he was 24. He remarried when he was 30, and is very happy, but still dreams of his first wife occasionally.

When you examine the timing of his life events, you see that the present rashes started relatively soon after the trauma of the loss of his first wife.

Revisiting the first short list, we find that *Nat Mur* fits the symptoms of the rash reasonably well, but fits the *never well since* situation in this case perfectly. *Nat Mur* is often used as a remedy to treat deep and unresolved grief.

This prescription would treat the patient on all levels – mental, emotional and physical – and could be expected to treat the true cause of the rash, rather than just the resulting physical symptoms.

This type of example is repeated again and again in the clinic, of course with differences in symptoms and timing. But the central point remains clear; we must treat the cause not the result to provide a true cure. In this, we act totally differently to pharmaceutical medicine, which sees the removal of superficial symptoms as being the goal.

Homoeopaths see suppression of superficial symptoms as one of the major causative factors in creating and worsening chronic disease. That is why we treat the patient, not the disease.

8 - The Most Similar Remedy

The *Law of Similars* requires us to find a remedy whose symptoms are very similar to the symptoms of the patient. In practice, a number of remedies will be closely similar. In theory one remedy should stand out as being the most similar – and it is called the *similimum*.

The ideal is to find the *similimum*, but we know in practice that a number of similar remedies can also assist the patient to heal.

To find an effective similar remedy we need to match the symptoms that are most significant in the patient, with similar symptoms in the remedy picture.

There are in fact four different types of *similimum*. They are:

1. The Symptom Similimum. This is the remedy that most closely matches the simple listing of individual symptoms. It is found by using methods 3 and 4 in Chapter 6.

2. The Aetiological Similimum. Aetiology = cause. So, this is the remedy that most closely relates to a stress that has caused the patient's symptom picture to permanently change. Some common aetiologies are loss of a loved one, a relationship break-up, major financial loss, being sacked from work, a severe infectious disease, vaccination, and so on. Homoeopathy has special remedies which assist in the removal of the unresolved stress or trauma, and allow the *Vital Force* to resume the healing process.

3. The Constitutional Similimum. This is the remedy that most closely matches the constitutional symptom picture. It is found by using method 5 in Chapter 6.

4. The Miasmic Similimum. This is the remedy that most closely matches the patient's active miasm. It is found by using method 6 in Chapter 6.

So it is possible to find a number of similar remedies.

Our eventual aim should be to find a single remedy that fits the symptom similimum, the constitutional similimum, as well as the miasmic similimum.

This is indeed possible, but generally will only happen when all the suppressed traumas that the patient has suffered over their life have been fully resolved or healed.

When we reach this point, we will have a remedy that will take the patient through to their highest possible level of health. This is a form of prescribing that requires great skill and experience and would be beyond beginners. However, it is good to know the eventual goal.

In the meantime, finding the symptom similimum, and prescribing it in an appropriate potency and frequency, can provide safe and effective relief. If a person has problems that don't readily respond to basic treatments, then the help of an experienced homoeopath should be sought.

9 - Selection of Dose – Potency, and Frequency of Repetition

Some practitioners believe that selecting a similar remedy is not too difficult, but that the really challenging questions come when we have to choose the ideal dose, i.e. the most similar remedy administered in the ideal potency and frequency of repetition.

It is hard to find consistent guidelines in the homoeopathic literature – there are high potency prescribers, low potency prescribers, and those who use every potency available. And of course, there is also disagreement as to what is a high and a low potency.

To give you a guide, the following potency ranges would be agreed by many Australian homoeopaths (although in Europe 30c is regarded as a high potency):

Low Potency - 3x to 12c
Medium Potency - 30c, 200c
High Potency - M, 10M
Very High Potency - 50M and above.

Figure 9.1 shows *7 Golden Rules* that can be followed when deciding what potency and frequency to use – they are very simple, but very effective to help you to avoid causing unnecessary aggravations which may result if the wrong potency and frequency are used.

The reason for the line is to show that the top 4 rules are "other things being equal". The lower 3 are for exceptions to the general rule.

For example, you may have a patient who is deeply unwell, with some severe health problems. You may have found a remedy that is an extremely close match to the patient's symptoms. So Rule 1 would suggest that a high potency be used, and Rule 3 would suggest that it be given infrequently.

However, if the patient is very weak and debilitated, it is most unwise to give a high potency. This is where Rule 5 comes in, and in this case a low potency would be used. Rule 4 would then direct that the remedy be given regularly.

Figure 9.1: The 7 Golden Rules of Potency and Dose

1. The more similar the remedy, the higher the potency.
2. The less similar the remedy, the lower the potency.
3. The higher the potency, the fewer doses needed.
4. The lower the potency the more doses needed.

---

5. The more severe the pathology, the lower the potency.
6. The more hypersensitive the patient, the lower the potency and frequency.
7. If in doubt, start low and work up higher.

These *7 Golden Rules* are different from what some practitioners would give as guidelines.

For example, some homoeopaths believe that low potencies should be used for physical conditions, when treating young people, and for acute conditions. They also claim that high potencies should be used for mental/emotional conditions.

As you can see, the *7 Golden Rules* result in different guidelines. High potencies should be used for acute and physical conditions if the similimum is strong and if the patient is robust and stable. They can be safely used for infants if similar and if the infant is generally healthy. Also, it is appropriate to use low potencies in mainly mental/emotional cases if the patient is weak or unstable, as the earlier example demonstrated.

But the key guideline in all cases is - **fit the prescription to the patient.** This applies not only to the selection of the most similar remedy, but also the potency and frequency used. Never be inflexible. Always be prepared to vary potency and frequency if the patient's condition requires it.

Table 9.2 shows some possible combinations of potency and frequency. Remember, **this is a guide only** for new prescribers. Your practitioner may use higher or lower potencies according to their own experience.

Some homoeopaths always use the same set of questions in case taking, always analyse the cases in the same way, always use high or low potencies, and always begin with the same frequency of repetition.

I believe such practices take away from one of the key advantages of homoeopathy stated earlier – the fact that it individualises each case to select the best possible remedy and dose for the patient.

Table 9.2: A Guide to Potency and Frequency

In Acute/Emergency Cases
30c or 200c every hour to every 3 hours. Reduce frequency as the symptoms improve.

In Moderately Severe Cases
30c once or twice a week.

In Chronic or Constitutional Cases
If debilitated - 6c daily, or 30c once or twice a week.
If robust - 30c to 1000c (M), depending on how similar the remedy is to the patients symptoms (give 30c weekly, give 200c or M every 2-4 weeks).

Selecting the perfect combination of potency and frequency is something only really learned from experience. But even experienced practitioners at times get caught out, particularly with hypersensitive patients. What can happen is a temporary aggravation of symptoms, which generally pass in time.

However, if you begin with either a 30c or a 200c, and in non-emergency cases give a single dose and wait for say a week, you will minimise the chance of aggravating the patient. If you find that there is improvement, but it does not last, give the remedy more often. If there is an improvement which does last, then delay giving the second dose.

Never repeat the dose during either an aggravation of symptoms or an improvement of symptoms. These are only happening because the remedy is working, so wait until the previous dose seems to have lost its effect, then repeat.

In emergency or acute conditions, the rules are slightly different. If, for example, a child has a high fever, you may give a dose of Belladonna 200 every 30 to 60 minutes. If there is no apparent response to the remedy after 2 or 3 doses, then you need to re-evaluate the remedy. It may be that the symptoms really did fit Aconite better. In these cases, you learn very quickly whether you have made a good choice.

If you follow the above guidelines, you will cause very few aggravations, and help many people to resolve their health problems, IF you choose a similar remedy to their complaints.

Appendix 7: Other resources by Dr Isaac Golden

Isaac Golden
PUBLICATIONS

Other books written and published by Dr Isaac Golden PhD, as at 30.8.2023
(Quantity discounts are available on request)

BOOKS ON HOMŒOPROPHYLAXIS

Immunisation Options for Parents Who Care. 2015
A small booklet to assist parents who are considering immunisation options, but want guidance through the mass of often conflicting information available in the media and on the internet.
$14.00 inc p&p to Victoria (additional p&p overseas, add $6.00)

The Complete Practitioners Manual of Homoeoprophylaxis. 2017
This book aims to provide homeopaths, as well as practitioners of any modality and students with a complete grounding in the topic. It contains comprehensive instructions how to implement both short-term and long-term HP programs, a thorough presentation of the evidentiary base of HP as well as an in-depth discussion of its philosophical underpinnings. This is the most comprehensive resource currently available internationally on the challenging topic of homeopathic immunisation. It is the accepted reference work on this topic. Whilst it is a practitioner's manual, parents who want to thoroughly research every aspect of homœoprophylaxis would find the material accessible, even if challenging. It includes all the responses from parents who used my HP program from 1986 to 2004 reporting reactions to the program plus the general effect of using the program on their children.
$44.00 inc p&p to Victoria (additional p&p overseas, add $8.00).

Vaccination & Homoeoprophylaxis? A Review of Risks and Alternatives. 7th edition, 2010.
This is a complete rewrite of the 6th edition, to improve readability, with updating of references in all sections. A new Section on the massive Cuban

HP intervention has been added. Examines the risks and benefits of vaccination, with a full discussion of the homoeopathic alternative. Includes details of Isaac's research over 25 years, including his Doctoral studies, and the history of the homoeopathic alternative. The main reference book for parents and practitioners researching the area for the first time. A4 size, 262 pages. $53.00 inc p&p (additional p&p overseas, add $8.00)

Homœoprophylaxis - A Fifteen Year Clinical Study: A Statistical Review of the Efficacy and Safety of Long-Term Homœoprophylaxis. 2004. An in-depth statistical analysis of 2,342 responses from parents whose children used my homœoprophylaxis program from 1986-2003. Includes written responses from parents describing reactions and diseases. Also data from 4-year General Health Study on long-term health, comparing effects of different methods of immunisation. A4 size, 150 pages. $34.00 inc p&p (additional postage overseas $9.00-$16.00).

Homœoprophylaxis-A Practical and Philosophical Review. 4th edition.2007. Examines the philosophical and practical arguments for and against homœoprophylaxis. A book for practitioners who are evaluating their options, and the points for and against using homoeopathic option. A5 size.
$18.00 inc p&p (add: interstate $2. 00, overseas $6. 00).

SIMPLE HOMOEOPATHIC PRESCRIBING

Australian Homoeopathic Home Prescriber - Part 1 - Treatment of Simple Everyday Conditions.3rd edition. 2007. A very simple, uncomplicated prescriber for parents. Quick and easy to use. Used by Martin & Pleasance in their First Aid kits. A5 size.
$14.00 inc p&p.

Australian Homoeopathic Home Prescriber - Part 2 - A Simple Materia Medica of Common Remedies With Repertory. 2001. An easy to read Materia Medica of common first-aid remedies, with a very simple, uncomplicated Repertory for parents- Quick and easy to use. A5 size

$16.00 inc p&p.

Australian Homoeopathic Home Prescriber - Part 3 – Basic Homoeopathy. 2006. A very simple, uncomplicated explanation of homoeopathic prescribing. Quick and easy to use.
A5 size. 13.00 inc p&p.
For the 3 books above add $15.00 for overseas postage.

DETAILED HOMOEOPATHIC BODY-SYSTEM PRESCRIBING

Homoeopathic Body-System Prescribing - A Practical Workbook of Sector Remedies. 2nd Ed. 2002. Homoeopathic analysis of major diseases from every body system. A major rewrite of this manual has just been completed. The 2nd Edition of the Workbook 10 new diseases, and substantially reworks 29 diseases that were in the 1ST edition A4 size. 420 pages. $66.00 inc. p&p (overseas post p.o.a.).

NEW DEVELOPMENTS IN HOMOEOPATHY

Homoeopathic Treatment of the Energy Bodies - Traditional Strategies And New Developments. 2002.
Homoeopathic medicines are energetic substances that interact with the energy bodies of the patient. An explanation of the bodies is given. The healing models of homoeopathy and theosophy are compared, and integrated. A new approach to remove negative material in the energy bodies of patients is introduced, using new equipment called the *Auric Replicator*- The use of potentised medicines in both chronic and acute cases is discussed B5 size, 99 pages.

Currently out of print

Visit our web page at www.homstudy.net

EDUCATION IN HOMOEOPATHY AND NATURAL MEDICINE

(1) Correspondence Courses written and supervised by Dr Isaac Golden, and now taught by Isaac's daughter Leiah Golden taught through the Australasian College of Hahnemannian Homoeopathy

Visit our web pages at https://www.homstudy.net/ACHHCOURSES/

An Intermediate Course in Homoeopathic Medicine
This course is designed for those who wish to learn how to prescribe accurately for the basic health problems of their family or friends. It gives credits for the Professional course if students continue with their studies. The 6 Tutorials are understandable and practical. The cost of $360.00 (inc. books) is spread over the 1ength of the course. Suitable for parents, students, or therapists who want a basic knowledge of practical homoeopathy.

Certificate Courses in Homeopathy
Two certificate courses for those who want to extend their studies.

An Introductory Course in Natural Medicine
This three Tutorial course introduces students to the use of herbal medicine, homoeopathy, flower essences, tissue salts, diet, and colour healing. A simple, "how to do it" course.

(2) On-Line Courses in Homoeopathy and Natural Medicine, written and supervised by Dr Isaac Golden, and taught through the Homeopathic International Online College

(3) Web based courses in Homoeoprophylaxis for parents and for practitioners, plus a practitioner's course in treating vaccine injured children as well as a course on Covid prevention and treatment.

See https://www.homstudy.net/natural-immunisation-research/ and https://www.homstudy.net/isaac-golden-education/

CONTACT: P.O. Box 695. Gisborne. Victoria. 3437. Australia.
Ph. (03) 5427 0880. Email: admin@homstudy.net

INDEX

Made in United States
Cleveland, OH
26 September 2026

44828275R00136